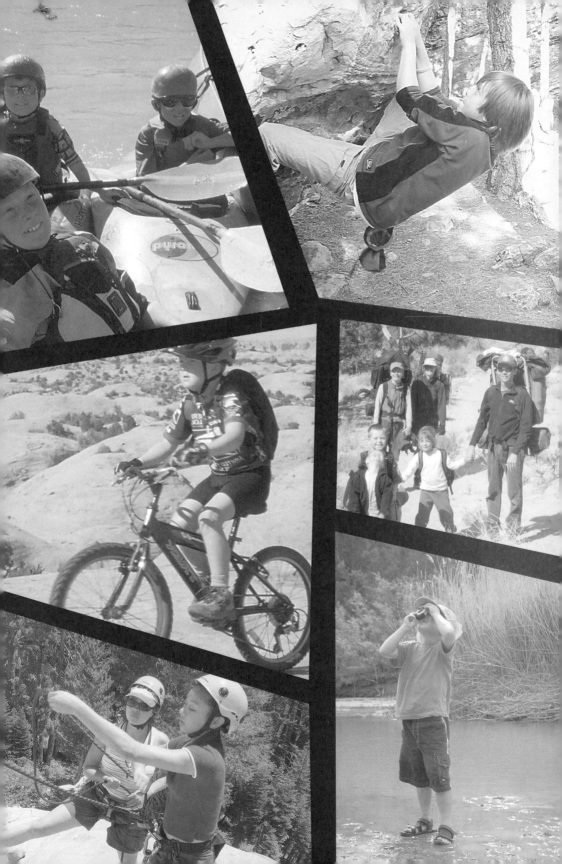

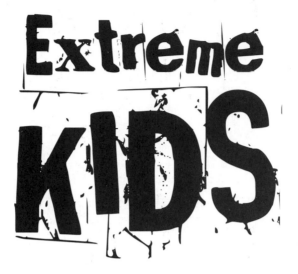

Extreme KIDS

how to connect with your children through today's extreme (and not so extreme) outdoor sports

Scott Graham

 WILDERNESS PRESS · BERKELEY, CA

Extreme Kids: how to connect with your children through today's
extreme (and not so extreme) outdoor sports

1st EDITION January 2006

Copyright © 2006 by Scott Graham

Front cover photos copyright © 2006 by (clockwise from top left):
   Scott Graham, Scott Graham, Nick Wilkes, Jackson Kayak,
   Scott Graham
Back cover photos copyright © 2006 by Scott Graham (bottom left)
   and GirlVentures (top right)
Interior photos by Scott Graham, except for those credited on page 282
Cover and book design: Lisa Pletka
Book editor: Eva Dienel

ISBN-13: 978-0-89997-373-9
ISBN-10: 0-89997-373-6
UPC 7-19609-97373-7

Manufactured in the United States of America

Published by: **Wilderness Press**
                1200 5th Street
                Berkeley, CA 94710
                (800) 443-7227; FAX (510) 558-1696
                info@wildernesspress.com
                www.wildernesspress.com

Visit our website for a complete listing of our books and for ordering
information.

For Sue, Taylor, and Logan

Acknowledgments

My sincere thanks go to the many parents, guides, and instructors who willingly shared their stories, expertise, advice, and photographs with me during the research phase of this book.

My thanks also go to Roslyn Bullas of Wilderness Press for championing the idea for *Extreme Kids*; to Eva Dienel, this book's talented and assiduous editor; and to Lisa Pletka, who incorporated into her design of *Extreme Kids* the same vision of fun with kids I had in mind while writing it.

Cast of Kids

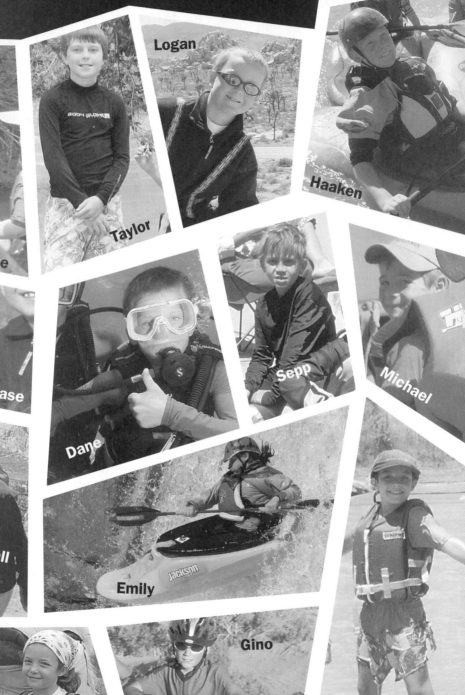

Logan

Haaken

Alicia Rose

Taylor

Chase

Dane

Sepp

Michael

Kendall

Emily

Gino

Carly

Colin

Contents

Preface

Snow Caving with a Preschooler

The glimmer of an idea struck me when my oldest son, Taylor, was coming up on his 5th birthday. I made the mistake, as I often do, of giving voice to my notion before I'd fully thought it through.

It was late winter. Taylor was playing blocks with his younger brother, Logan, then 2, on the living room floor. That winter, my wife, Sue, and I had spent as much time as possible outdoors with the boys near our Durango, Colorado, home in the southern Rockies. We had sledded, gotten both boys up and skiing, and snowshoed with Logan in a child carrier and Taylor in little-kid snowshoes. Still, there were only so many hours a 4-year-old and 2-year-old could spend out in the cold. For the most part, while Sue worked that winter, my at-home-dad duties had kept me indoors. I was beginning to feel the full weight of being housebound.

"I was just thinking," I said, addressing Taylor. He paused from his block work and eyed me. "Maybe we could go snow caving for your birthday."

His little brow crinkled. "What's snow caving?" he asked.

I described the glory of the endeavor in elaborate detail, the concept of building our own truly wondrous fort in the snow and then sleeping in it—really sleeping in it!—overnight. I gushed about the glittering ice crystals, the hot chocolate by candlelight, the stars in the clear night sky. By the time I finished, Taylor's eyes glowed with excitement.

"That sounds GREAT!" he shouted.

Logan raised a small clenched fist in solidarity.

It was then that the first little "uh-oh" sounded from deep inside me. How in the world was I going to pull off the fun-filled adventure I'd just described to Taylor?

In our lives B.C. (Before Children) Sue and I had climbed and camped at altitude in the Andes, the Canadian Rockies, and the Himalayas. We'd winter camped and snow caved in this country as well. As Taylor and Logan returned to their blocks, I recalled our many high-mountain camps. Though those camps had made possible the climbing Sue and I loved, three words described every one of them: dank, cold, and uncomfortable—not quite the scene that would appeal to a 5-year-old.

But now I was committed. I took a deep breath and began planning our overnighter.

When Taylor's birthday came, I drove with Taylor and Logan to the top of Coalbank Pass, a half an hour north of town. Pulling Logan behind me on a snow saucer, I snowshoed with Taylor to a wind-loaded pile of snow in a small clearing among firs a hundred yards off the highway. There, Taylor and I set to work crafting our masterpiece in

advance of Logan's
nap time.

Taylor lasted about five minutes with his tiny plastic shovel, and then he set about keeping a fast-chilling Logan occupied with songs and games of mittened patty-cake. I dug with a vengeance, aware that at any moment, Logan, rendered immobile in so many layers of fleece and trapped in his snow saucer, might decide to wail about his situation. Just in time, I managed to shovel out a small cave that included a sleeping platform and a candle nook, then I scooped up Logan, and we all slogged back to the car.

Logan napped during our drive home while Taylor chattered nonstop, weighing his anticipation against his trepidation about the night that lay ahead of him. When Sue got home from work, we celebrated Taylor's birthday as a family with an early supper and cake. Afterward, Taylor and I headed back up the pass, arriving just before dark.

We snowshoed to the cave as daylight disappeared and the cold came on. I carried an expeditionary pack filled with four sleeping bags, four pads, and layer upon layer of warm clothing, while Taylor carried a sack containing snacks, a thermos of hot chocolate, and a candle lantern.

Arriving at our spot, we slid into the cave, lit the lantern, and settled into our doubled bags, which lay atop doubled pads and inside an unerected two-man tent that served as a moisture barrier. After oatmeal cookies and

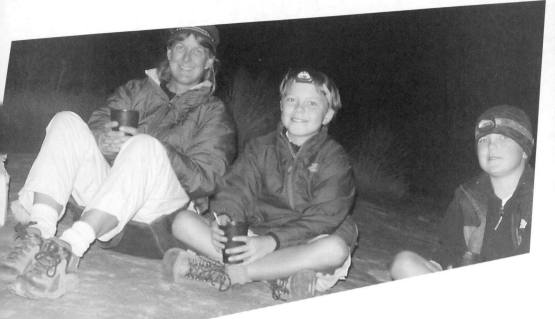

hot cocoa, we left the cave to stare up at the stars for a short, freezing minute, and then we shimmied back inside.

The excitement of the day was all that was necessary to send Taylor into a deep sleep minutes after we blew out the candle. I checked my watch. Not even 8. Lying on my back, I noticed for the first time the lumpiness of the sleeping platform beneath me.

Taylor slept soundly for the next 11 hours, during which time I managed a few hours of fitful sleep and a lot more time spent second-guessing my idea to take my preschooler snow caving.

Morning came slowly. The cave turned gray, then brightened. I rolled over, bumping Taylor. Nothing. I gave him another 30 minutes, and then bumped him again. He stirred and awoke.

The wide-eyed look of pride and accomplishment that swept across Taylor's face as soon as he remembered where he was and what he'd done was as gratifying as anything I'd experienced to that point as a parent. I swelled with reflected pride and slapped him a frosty high five.

We packed up, returned to the car, and were home for breakfast with Sue and Logan 45 minutes later.

In the years since, our night in the snow cave has come to be a touchstone event against which the many other outdoor experiences Sue and I seek out with our sons are measured. That night's freshness of adventure, the way Taylor at preschool age found the extreme in what many adults might consider a run-of-the-mill (not to mention uncomfortable) outdoor experience has driven my family's ongoing search for the new and different in the backcountry.

The fruits of that search for adventure with our children are at the heart of this book, as are the tales of adventure from many other parents and kids. All the stories included in these pages, all the how to's and where to's and when to's and why to's, are aimed at giving you the opportunity to experience similar life-affirming outdoor adventures with your own children—and at assuring you and your kids have a terrific time while doing so.

Scott Graham
Durango, Colorado
January 2006

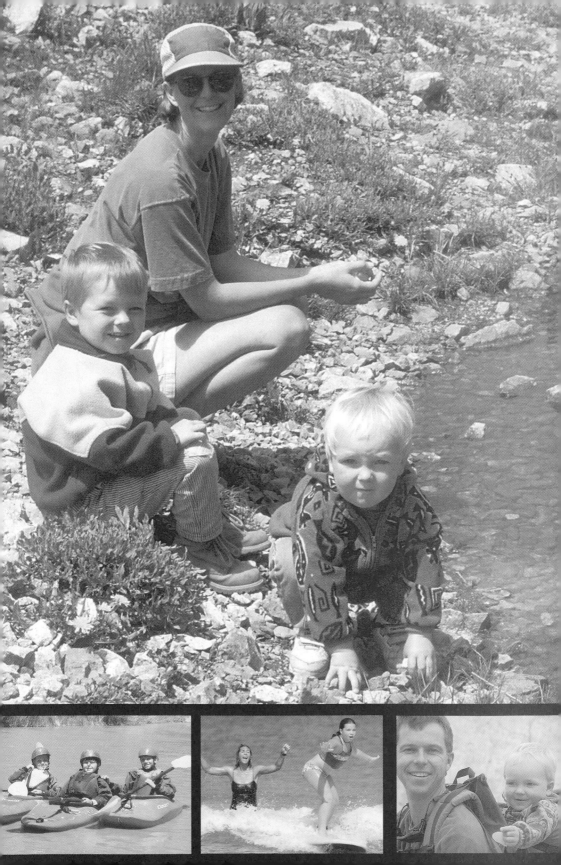

PART ONE

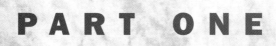

KIDS
OUTDOORS

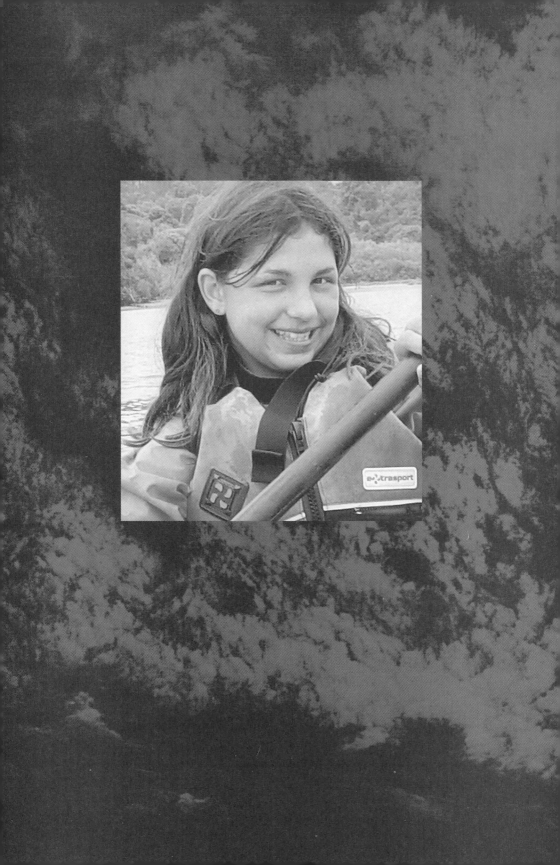

1 Extreme Fun

A few years ago, John and Mary Mummery left their son Colin, then 6, aboard a dive boat in the care of the boat's crew off the coast of Little Cayman Island in the Caribbean. They did so while they dove on a coral reef 100 feet below the ocean's surface. Near the end of their dive, John and Mary glanced up to see a horrifying sight: The dive boat, settling stern first in the water, was sinking fast.

Before they could ascend, the boat plunged past them to the seabed—fortunately with no sign of Colin or anyone else still on board. John and Mary found Colin on a neighboring dive boat when they reached the surface.

"That was when we decided it was safer to have our kids with us, doing the things we like to do, than to leave them behind," Mary says today with a wry grin.

Colin signed up for the Professional Association of Diving Instructors (PADI) Seal Team kids' scuba program as soon as he turned 8, the minimum age to begin PADI's classes. At 10, again the minimum age, Colin passed PADI's open-water certification test. As of this writing, Colin, at age 11, is an accomplished diver, having recently completed 25 dives with his parents during a return visit to the Caymans.

These days, John and Mary are busy with Colin and their three other preadolescent children, enjoying a host of other outdoor pursuits, from skiing and river running to mountain biking and bodyboarding.

"They're all great," says Mary of the various outdoor sports she and John take on with their brood, "because they're all fun. Plus, depending on the kids' ages, even the simplest sports are plenty challenging for them."

Why Extreme?

Fun and challenging. Those two words explain why more and more parents are joining the Mummerys in taking on so-called extreme outdoor sports with their preadolescent children. But what, exactly, does extreme mean when it comes to kids?

Many of the outdoor family adventures detailed in this book measure up as fully extreme on the adrenaline scale. Just as many do not. But all are fully extreme to

the right child at the right age with the right parent when measured on the emotional scale.

That's the definition of extreme used in these pages: For kids, extreme outdoor sports are any and all of those that children find extreme.

Snow caving with a preschooler, dayhiking with a kindergartner, scuba diving with a preadolescent—how extreme each activity is lies in the age and psyche of each participant.

Simply put, extreme kids are those who explore the outdoors in ways that are fun and exciting for themselves and themselves alone.

Consider rock climbing. For one child, the sport may consist of successfully sending a demanding route to a point high atop a vertical face. Another child of exactly the same age may find plenty of excitement in the sport simply by making a few friction moves on a sloped slab of rock a few feet off the ground. In both cases, the children are participating in what for them is fully extreme rock climbing.

Given that broad definition, as much as extreme means fun through challenge, it in no way means unsafe.

The aim of outdoor adventuring is exhilaration for you and your kids, yes, but only within the limits of each outdoor adventurer—and, just as important, only within the limits of the person leading a given outdoor adventure, whether that leader is you, a friend, or a professional guide.

Extreme is about excitement, but in a fully safe manner. It's about personal growth through new accomplishments. It's *not* about defying death. Just the opposite, in fact. Extreme is about reveling in life. It's about all the fun that's out there just waiting for you and your kids to have together.

As much as extreme means fun through challenge, it in no way means unsafe.

For You

In many cases when it comes to outdoor sports, the kids are out of the house while their parents remain behind—often at their parents' urging. While the kids are throwing ends in their playboats, mastering cross-body dynos on bouldering routes, and hucking mega wheelie drops on their mountain bikes, their parents are nowhere to be seen.

It needn't be that way. It's easy to participate in a whole range of today's hottest outdoor sports right alongside your kids—and have a blast doing it.

This book is for you if you're a parent and an old hand at the outdoors, and you're curious about the many family adventures available to you as your children grow up. This book is also for you if you want to discover the world of the outdoors for the first time with your children in ways that will engross and excite them (and you as well) rather than elicit yawns and disgusted rolls of the eyes.

If you're new to outdoor adventuring, *Extreme Kids* is designed to help you get started with your children. If you're an old hand at outdoor action sports, *Extreme Kids* will help you understand the unique needs of children when it comes to outdoor sports and adventure, and how best to introduce your kids to the outdoor sports you already pursue. This book also outlines other sports you

This Book is for You If...

■ You're a **parent and an old hand at the outdoors**, and you're curious about the many family adventures available to you as your children grow up, and the ages at which it's possible to try various outdoor sports with your kids.

■ You want to **discover the world of the outdoors for the first time with your children** in ways that will engross and excite them rather than elicit yawns and disgusted rolls of the eyes.

might want to try with your children, and directs you to the best resources, from outfitters to kid-specific gear, for those activities.

Whether you're new to outdoor sports or an experienced outdoor adventurer, *Extreme Kids* will enable you to confidently take your kids on any of the outdoor sports and adventures detailed in the chapters that follow, including surfing, peak bagging, canyoneering, mountain biking, and whitewater kayaking, to name only a few.

The convergence of fun and challenge for the entire family is unique to outdoor action sports. While team sports relegate parents to the role of shuttle drivers or coaches, the outdoor sports detailed in this book offer fun and challenge for you and your kids alike. They do so, that is, provided you choose to join your kids in these outdoor adventures rather than send them off to try such pursuits on their own.

For years, my wife, Sue, and I enjoyed the outdoors as a child-free couple, calmly and sedately. We perfected our favorite backpacking meals and figured out how best to transport wine into the backcountry. We climbed and trekked overseas. Closer to home, we telemark skied, canoed, and sea kayaked.

When our sons, Taylor and Logan, came along, we continued to enjoy the outdoors with them in tow. We shortened our summer back-packing trips and toured the winter back-country on skis with our boys in child carriers.

But things changed as our boys grew older. First came Taylor's and my snow-caving adventure. Before another year passed, Sue and I found ourselves pandering to Taylor's natural inclination toward anything and everything in the outdoors that his little-kid mind considered new, radical, or cool. And we found ourselves loving everything we tackled with him.

Over the last few years, Sue and I have par-ticipated first with Taylor, then with Logan in increasingly adventurous outdoor activities—all in extremely safe ways. The results have been fantas-tic. Taylor and Logan have grown to love the outdoors, and Sue and I have grown to love doing wild things in the wilds with them—including a number of new sports we'd never have experienced if not for our kids. Best of all, we've gotten to know our boys intimately, and they have us, through our mutual participation in outdoor fun of the most invigorating kind.

Extreme Kids is a compilation of what Sue and I, other parents, and outdoor-sport instructors have learned from participating with, coaching, and guiding kids and families in the world of hard-core and not-so-hard-core outdoor action sports.

Throughout *Extreme Kids*, parents tell the stories of their involvement with their children in the world of outdoor sports—involvement that results in close family relationships at a time in our society when the very idea of "family time" is at risk. Through those stories, you'll learn of countless possibilities for enjoying the natural world with your own children in ways that are truly extreme, or that aren't too extreme at all—but constitute terrific family outdoor adventures nonetheless.

Included as well are descriptions and contact information for more than 125 of the coolest, farthest-out-there trips and activities you may want to undertake with your children, all with an eye toward realizing the many benefits of seeking out adventure in the outdoors as a family. Those benefits include:

■ Forging solid connections with your kids that will last a lifetime.

■ Instilling safety consciousness in your kids early on in their lives.

■ Infusing your kids with self-confidence that will serve them well as they grow up.

■ Most important, simply having huge amounts of fun in the outdoors with your kids while they're young.

Reader's Guide

The first section of *Extreme Kids* is devoted to the overall topic of outdoor sports and adventuring with your kids. In it, you'll learn about the tremendous boom in family outdoor adventuring, the reasons so many parents are tackling outdoor action sports with their kids, and how best to get started outdoor adventuring with your own kids.

The idea of "extreme" as it relates to youngsters also is explored in detail in the first section of *Extreme Kids*, as is the all-important topic of safety. And a full chapter is devoted to the often vexing gear decisions you'll face upon entering the world of outdoor adventuring with your kids.

The final two sections of *Extreme Kids* are devoted to detailed descriptions of the outdoor action sports best suited to families. The first of those two sections covers sports pursued on land, and the second covers water sports. Within each section, the chapters are arranged based roughly on difficulty level.

Each chapter on an individual sport contains a description of the sport itself, the potential for family participation in that sport, and personal stories from parents who have tried the sports with their kids and/or from outfitters and guides who lead family adventures in that particular sport. Each sport chapter ends with a detailed description of specific possibilities—places, outfitters, and ideas—you may want to explore further with your kids.

Web addresses are included for each possibility. Where necessary, keywords you'll need to click once you reach an initial home page are included. For national park websites in particular, you'll need to click on the keywords "Activities" and "Plan Your Visit" to reach detailed information about backcountry adventures in specific parks.

A "Basics" box at the beginning of each sport chapter summarizes the key points regarding each sport, enabling you to quickly narrow your focus to the sports that interest you most.

Lastly, makes and models of various types of kid-specific outdoor gear are described throughout *Extreme Kids*. Outdoor gear manufacturers change model names and styles as fast as supermodels change hair colors. It's worth noting, then, that some of the make and model information included in this book will be out of date the minute the book goes to press. It's just as important to note, however, that the basic why-buy-this-or-that discussion accompanying the various descriptions of kid gear will hold true for years to come.

The convergence of fun and challenge for the entire family is unique to outdoor action sports.

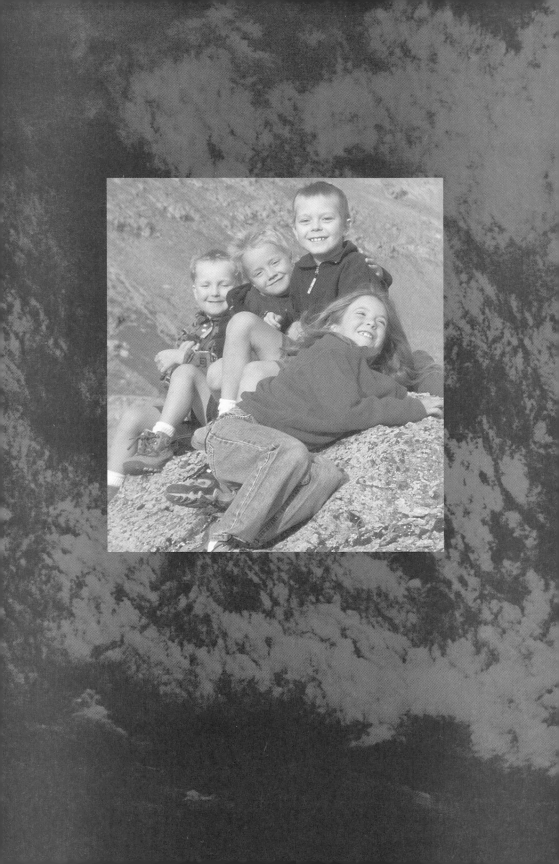

2 The Boom in Family Outdoor Adventuring

Eleven-year-old scuba diver Colin Mummery isn't alone in his desire and ability to participate as a youngster in an outdoor sport once considered the sole province of teenagers and adults. Nor are Colin's parents, Mary and John Mummery, alone in sharing their love of outdoor sports with their preadolescent son. Many parents today are turning their kids on to outdoor sports that until recently were considered too radical for youngsters, and outdoor sport manufacturers and outfitters are taking note.

In 2004, world-champion freestyle kayaker Eric Jackson, the father of a daughter and son eager to emulate their dad, sniffed a trend in the making and began producing the Fun 1, a tiny whitewater kayak for paddlers who weigh 80 pounds or less. Rock Island, Tennessee-based Jackson Kayak sold more Fun 1s the first six months following the boat's introduction than the company expected to sell the entire first year, and the Fun 1 has sold steadily since. (To whit: I recently spotted a 3-year-old paddling a Fun 1 around a local pool with his mom and dad.)

When it comes to other sports such as rock climbing, cycling, and trekking, the trend toward kids and families is just as strong.

Eastern Mountain Sports climbing school manager David Kelly reports that the number of children and families signing up for one of EMS's many rock climbing courses has been growing at a phenomenal rate. In 2005, EMS rolled out its Family Climbing Camp at all six of its Northeast climbing locations. The company did so after a pilot run in 2004 at EMS's New Hampshire headquarters site proved extraordinarily successful. EMS accepts climbers as young as 4 for its family courses.

Many parents today are turning their kids on to outdoor sports that until recently were considered too radical for youngsters.

Moab, Utah-based Western Spirit Cycling Adventures introduced its first backcountry mountain biking trip for families in 2000. Today, Western Spirit offers eight family mountain biking adventures around the country, and those backcountry trips account for a full one-third of the outfitter's business. "We have families who have gone on all our trips and are just waiting for us to add more so they can go on those, too," says Western Spirit owner Ashley Korenblat. Children as young as 2, who tag along in pull-behind trailers, are welcome on the trips.

In northern New Mexico, Taos-based Wild Earth Llama Adventures' Stuart Wilde reports that "more and more and more" of the people he guides on wilderness llama pack trips are families with children. "It's up to 60 percent of my business now, and it's just not stopping," he says. Wilde has taken families with babies as young as three months on multiday journeys into the backcountry, and he has led kids as young as 5 up the area's 12,000- and 13,000-foot peaks.

The Genesis of the Outdoor-Sports Boom

Among teenagers and 20-somethings, the boom in fast-paced, or "extreme," outdoor sports began with the inception of ESPN's X Games in 1995. As the teen and young-adult audience for the X Games has grown in the years since, so, too, has participation in outdoor action sports by the same group. The Outdoor Industry Association reports, for example, that over the last few years, participation in playboat kayaking has increased 77 percent among those between the ages of 16 and 24, while telemark skiing is up more than 300 percent among the same age group. Even trail running, at the low end of the adrenaline scale, is up 30 percent.

The increase in participation by parents and pre-teens in outdoor sports has followed the boom among the teen and 20-something crowd. The families-with-kids boom is readily apparent in the travel arena. Larry Mogelonsky, executive director of the San Francisco-based Adventure Collection, an association of adventure tour operators, says many of the operators he represents have seen their bookings for families with children increase by more than 70 percent in the last few years.

From luxury adventure tours to low-cost camping trips, outfitted outdoor adventuring with children is popular. "What we're seeing on the outfitter end of things is that parents want a more intensive holiday for themselves and their kids," Mogelonsky says. "'Wherever we're going,' they're saying, 'we want to get the most out of it.'"

Donnie Dove owns Flagstaff, Arizona-based Canyon Rio Rafting, which runs trips for families on rivers in the Southwest. Dove points to the 9/11 attacks as a significant impetus for the increased family business Canyon Rio has seen since 2001. "Up to 9/11 we saw a decline in family multiday adventure trips," says Dove.

Before 9/11, Dove says, families were so busy with work and school and after-school activities that they could squeeze in only what Dove calls "sound-bite" experiences—half-day river trips and other short vacations. Parents didn't have time—or didn't make the time—for the longer, more experiential family trips of the sort Canyon Rio offers.

"After 9/11 there was a retrenching of values, of what it means to have children," Dove says. "The 9/11 attacks got people thinking about what they'll be leaving their kids with when they're gone."

The result has been a steady increase in family business for Canyon Rio, and for outdoor action sport outfitters across the board.

Bringing the Kids Along

The family outdoor industry is booming in part because of a parallel trend: Those people who grew up in the '60s, '70s, and '80s with the advent of backpacking, mountain biking, snowboarding, and other adventure sports now have kids that they'd like to bring along on their outdoor pursuits.

"The children of the outdoors have grown up," says Wild Earth Llamas' Wilde, referring to those of us who came of age during backpacking and camping boom of the last few decades. That boom followed the development of the first generation of lightweight camping and backpacking gear, and the publication of books like Edward Abbey's *Desert Solitaire* and Colin Fletcher's *The Man Who Walked Through Time*.

"We're parents now," says Wilde, "but we don't want to give up our passion and connection to the outdoor world. Instead, we want to share it with our kids."

This trend is easy to spot here in my hometown of Durango, Colorado. Durango, set between mountains and desert in far southwestern Colorado, long has been a mecca for outdoor athletes eager to mountain bike, ski, and climb— often all on the same day.

The outdoor athletes who were drawn to Durango a decade or two ago now have gray in their hair and children of their own—and they're taking their kids along on the pastimes that long have defined their lives. These days the trails around Durango teem with parents

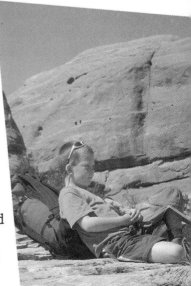

and kids mountain biking together. Moms and dads telemark with their children at the local ski area and in the backcountry in winter. In summer, the river through town is busy with parents and kids taking turns surfing waves and pulling play-hole tricks.

In New Mexico, Wilde and his wife, parents of a teenager and a preadolescent, have been exploring the outdoors with their offspring since shortly after their children were born. "It's been a beautiful thing," Wilde says with the wistful air of a parent watching his kids grow up too fast.

Wilde is quick to point out that sharing the wonders of the outdoors with children isn't limited to parents who were already outdoor-experienced before they had kids. Many of the parents in families Wilde takes into the backcountry have never before explored the outdoors. "For them, it's almost better," Wilde says of the first-timer parents, "because they're getting to experience it fresh along with their kids."

Western Spirit Cycling's Korenblat says that's a big reason why companies like hers are so popular. "We're here for everybody who can't get into the backcountry on their own," she says. "If you're coming in from Chicago or wherever, if you've never done anything in the backcountry before, we're here so that you can do it without you or your kids getting dehydrated or sunburned or injured."

Creating that possibility for parents and kids has led directly to the increase in family business Western Spirit has experienced since 2000, and to the similar increase in family business experienced by other outfitters.

The Adventure Collection's Mogelonsky says that the boom in adventure family travel is just beginning. He says tour operators should expect families to demand that the trips they sign up for be even more outdoor-action-oriented in the years ahead.

"Parents, obviously, drive the family-travel market," says Mogelonsky. "Today's parents have high expectations and they want great experiences, for themselves and their kids. That's a trend I see only growing stronger, regardless of whether parents are heading into the outdoors with outfitters or on their own."

Today's older outdoor athletes are taking their kids along on the pastimes that long have defined their lives.

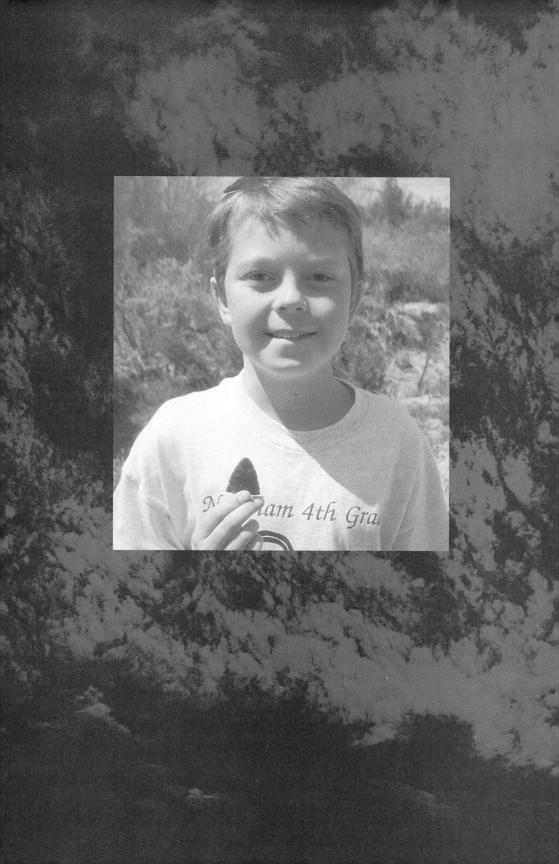

3

Why You Should Do It: The Practical Reasons

Every parent, guide, and outfitter who has participated with children in outdoor action sports has seen firsthand the many benefits that come from interacting with kids through those sports. The reasons for undertaking such sports with kids are many, they say with one voice, and they are real.

Long-time rock climbing guide and instructor Jon Ross of High Angle Adventures in eastern New York points out that outdoor action sports like climbing "foster a lot of the values parents are looking to convey to their kids—respect for dangerous situations, and a strong sense of accomplishment and self-esteem through character-building experiences."

Best of all, Ross notes, those values are instilled in ways that are totally fun for kids and parents alike—which is reason number one for undertaking outdoor action sports with your kids.

It's Fun

Like Sue and me, scuba diver Colin Mummery's parents, John and Mary, are adamant about seeking the new and different in the outdoors with their kids—all *four* of them.

John and Mary come by their stamina honestly. For kicks while living in Alaska, John scuba dived the seas off Anchorage in midwinter. He nearly died in a ferocious storm on the knife-edge summit ridge of Mt. Foraker in

17

the Alaska Range. Mary was raised canoeing the farthest reaches of northern Minnesota's Boundary Waters before becoming one of America's youngest-ever female commercial pilots.

It's their own history of adventurousness, John is quick to point out, that has made them so determined to share the outdoors in active ways with their children. "Basically,

Six Practical Reasons for Outdoor Adventuring with Your Kids

1. Most important: It's fun.

2. It's affordable.

3. You'll end up with incredibly capable kids.

4. It's (don't let the kids read this) educational.

5. You'll instill safety consciousness in your children early in their lives.

6. Your own life will be enriched.

it's fun," says John, who now lives with his family in Durango. "For us, it's not about how radical the stuff is we're doing with our kids, because, frankly, while much of what we do seems extreme to the kids, it's not really all that extreme from an adult point of view. It's really about being together as a family, about having a great time with our kids doing things in the outdoors we all like to do—and can do—together."

Part of the reason more parents are choosing to undertake outdoor action sports with their kids may well be the growing backlash against some of the un-fun aspects of team sports for youngsters.

After decades of exponential growth that began with the founding of Pop Warner football and Little League baseball in the 1930s, the Sporting Goods Manufacturers Association reports that participation in team sports by kids between the ages of 6 and 17 dropped significantly from 1990 to 2002, even while the number of children in America climbed by more than seven million. These days, adults in control of youngsters' team sports demand such single-minded devotion to their sports from such young ages that the dropout rate is up to 70 percent.

Like the Mummerys, more families are opting out of the Soccer Family scenario that requires kids as young as 5 to devote themselves year-round to a single sport and travel far from home on weekends for tournaments. Instead, they're pursuing activities together.

"The problem with travel teams is that you invariably end up farming your kids out to other families," Mary says. "For us, especially with four kids, we can't be at four different competitions in four different places at once. And we didn't have kids just so we could ship them away with other families—or to spend our family life traveling from city to city for yet another tournament."

The Mummerys use the outdoors to inject excitement into their family life. "The weekends are our time as a family," says John, who works as an oil-and-gas engineer. "But the only way it'll be that way is if the things we do on the weekends with our kids are fun—for them *and* for us."

In addition to one big scuba diving trip each year (which translates into a snorkeling trip for the younger ones), the Mummerys take their kids skiing, canoeing, and river running. They also car camp extensively, using

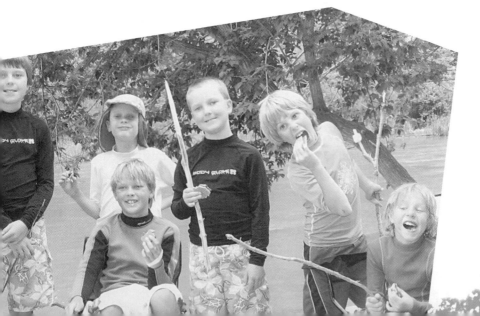

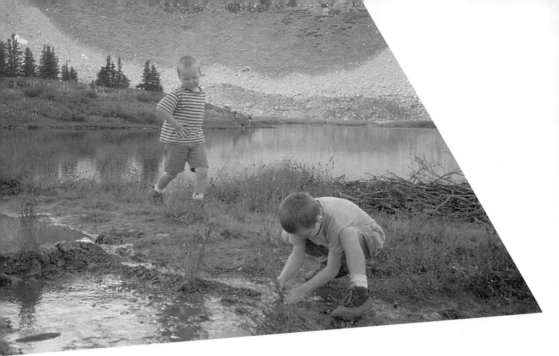

their campsites as bases for mountain biking, peak bagging, and short backpacking trips.

"Whatever we do, as long as it's in the outdoors, the kids have fun doing it, and we have fun with them," Mary says. "It really is just one big jungle gym out there."

It's Affordable

Virtually any outdoor adventure is far less expensive than a city-based family vacation, even if you need to buy or rent equipment to pull it off.

A do-it-yourself canoe trip in northern Minnesota's Boundary Waters Canoe Area Wilderness, for example, will run you only $50 a day per high-quality rental canoe from one of the many outfitters in the nearby town of Ely. For additional reasonable amounts, outfitters will broker an entry permit for you, shuttle you to your put-in and take-out points, and provide you with camping gear and pre-packaged meals for your journey.

If you and your kids tackle a day or multiday trip for which you already own all the gear and possess all the skills you need, the only costs will be for travel, food, and, if needed, permits.

Want a guided trip? You'll find that most outfitted outdoor adventures are comparable in cost to city vacations.

And if you want a guide or instructor but must keep finances in mind, a little searching on the internet—and in the "Possibilities" sections in each chapter in parts two and three of this book—will reveal numerous affordable and fun trips and courses offered by highly respected out-fitters and instructors who provide great experiences at reasonable prices.

As one example among thousands, Bear Valley, California-based Mountain Adventure Seminars offers full-day beginner rock climbing classes for families with children as young as 6 on crags in the Bay Area for only $50 per person, which makes a lesson well worth including as part of a vacation to San Francisco.

Guided outdoor adventures that involve camping as opposed to staying in hotels often are especially afford-able. Western Spirit's five-day family mountain biking trips, for example, are priced at $700 to $900 per person, including biking and camping equipment, shuttles, and all meals.

Perhaps the best thing about outdoor adventuring with children is that such adventures teach kids to think for themselves.

You'll End Up with Capable Kids

Perhaps the best thing about outdoor adventuring with children is that such adventures teach kids to think for themselves. When kids paddle their own kayaks down a river, it's up to them to choose the best route downstream. When they lead the way up a mountain, they decide how best to reach the summit. When they go off exploring from camp, they must note where they go and how to get back. All such demands, which are naturally placed on kids who engage in outdoor action sports, make them capable decision-makers—a skill that will serve them well for the rest of their lives.

Every outdoor guide and instructor I spoke with while researching this book noted how quickly children master the various outdoor sports they undertake, and how quickly they become capable of taking care of themselves and helping others as a result.

I've experienced that learned capability firsthand.

I pride myself on my own capabilities as a parent, and I think of myself as being especially conscientious when I'm entrusted with someone else's child. There was a day not long ago, however, when I found out just how incapable I can be, and, conversely, how capable are kids who have been raised participating in outdoor action sports.

Sue, Taylor, Logan, and I were on a three-day river trip with two other families. One family had a 7-year-old, Michael, who'd never kayaked. He asked if he could try out Logan's boat. I assured Michael's mother I would look after her son while he took Logan's kayak for a spin in the eddy alongside the beach where we'd made camp.

Kids who have been raised participating in outdoor action sports are incredibly capable.

While the other five adults relaxed on shore, I stood knee-deep in the river, watching Michael as he paddled an erratic course up and down the eddy. He remained within a few feet of the beach until a sudden gust of wind blew down the canyon. (Wind gusts had blasted down the canyon all afternoon, but I'd neglected to keep that fact in mind as I stood watch over Michael.)

Though the gust sent Michael skittering from the eddy into the main current, I wasn't worried. The river's current was fairly slow here, and the previous gusts had died away quickly. I was sure that as soon as this gust died down, Michael would be able to paddle back to shore. Besides, I didn't really want to get wet swimming out to retrieve him. I called out to Michael to paddle back toward me while I waited for the wind to let up. Trouble was, the wind *didn't* let up. Instead, it strengthened in intensity, blowing Michael farther from shore.

A quick glance to my left told me what I already knew: Michael was heading for a small rapid that piled against a low gray cliff about 100 yards downstream. The rapid wasn't life threatening, but it certainly wasn't something Michael needed to experience the first time he'd ever sat in a kayak.

I had to act. But what was I to do? I'd been dumb enough to set Michael loose in the eddy without tethering his boat to me with a length of rope. Now Michael was in the middle of the river and drifting farther away from me with each passing second, his face white, his eyes wide with fear.

Before I could act, two young kayakers from our group, Haaken, 11, and Sepp, 9, came to Michael's—and my—rescue. The boys, both experienced kayakers who had been messing around in the eddy in their boats, paddled out to Michael.

Haaken tried herding Michael's boat back toward the beach, but the wind was so strong he managed only to hold Michael in place. Haaken acted decisively as soon as he saw that he wasn't going to be able to return Michael to shore in Logan's boat.

"Jump in the water," he told Michael.

Michael obeyed immediately, diving into the river from the open cockpit of Logan's kayak.

"Grab the handle on the back of my boat," Haaken instructed in a calm voice.

Michael did as told and Haaken paddled back to shore through the wind, towing Michael behind him. Sepp, following, gathered up the paddle Michael had abandoned.

As for me? I was riveted by the scene of Haaken and Sepp capably coming to Michael's aid—so riveted, in fact, that I forgot about Logan's now-empty boat floating away downstream. Before my thoughts turned to it, there was a flash beside me as Sepp's mother, Sabina, dove into the water. She swam to Logan's kayak and side-stroked her way out of the current with the boat in her grasp, reaching shore just above the rapid.

At this point, I finally broke into action. I set down the beer I'd been holding, walked along the riverbank, and sheepishly helped Sabina carry Logan's boat back upstream. I returned to camp humbled and thoroughly impressed by Haaken and Sepp's ability to take stock of Michael's predicament, assess the alternatives, and carry out a plan that resulted in his quick return to shore.

Of course, much more than just participation in outdoor sports results in capable children like Haaken and Sepp. But nothing I know of does so quite as well.

"Kids on our trips have to look within themselves to see if they can actually do something," says Canyon Rio owner Donnie Dove, whose family river trips involve children paddling their own kayaks on the water, and rock climbing with ropes and harnesses on shore.

The result? Capable kids.

It's Educational

There's no better science instructor than the outdoors. Wind and river currents teach wave theory. Playing hard and eating lots of food afterward teaches energy consumption and replenishment, while putting on a jacket during a break along the trail teaches energy conservation.

Virtually every outdoor action sport has a built-in learning opportunity for kids. Dealing with thunderstorms or snow

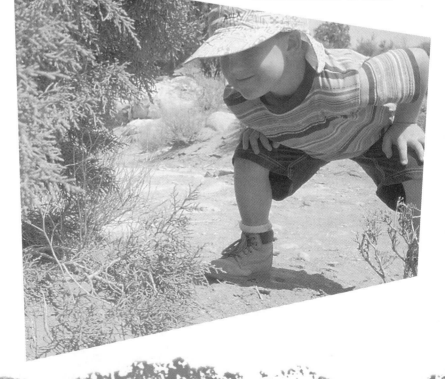

and cold teach children that even the best things in life involve hardship. The inevitable human dynamics of group trips, both good and bad, teach children social skills. Gathering firewood, setting up camps, preparing meals, washing dishes—all teach teamwork.

Guided family trips often include more overt forms of education.

"We try to teach the kids about the area they're visiting, but without it seeming like we're really teaching them," says Western Spirit Cycling's Korenblat of the outfitter's family mountain biking trips. "We try to keep it fun."

One evening during Western Spirit's Grand Canyon family mountain biking trip, for example, guides use tarps of various colors laid atop one another to illustrate the canyon's rock layers. Parents rise up from beneath the tarps to demonstrate the geologic processes of uplift and fault creation. Korenblat reports that kids on the Grand Canyon trips delight in seeing their parents as forces of nature, and as a result they're a bit more attuned to their surroundings than they were before watching the skit.

Suzanne Strazza and her husband have taken their two sons on desert river trips with other families since their boys were 3 and 1. Strazza says the river trips have been educational even for very young children.

"Our boys know to drink plenty of fluids when it's sunny, and to wet their baseball caps in the river when it's hot," she says. "Before they could add 2 and 2, they could help stake out our tent when it was windy and put on the fly when it was cloudy. And, most important, they knew to zip the door shut to keep the scorpions out."

> **Virtually every outdoor action sport has a built-in learning opportunity for kids.**

You'll Instill Safety Consciousness in Your Kids

I've often heard parents express concern that if kids are introduced to outdoor action sports as preadolescents, they will go on to try ever more extreme versions of those sports as they enter their teens and 20s—and so will be more likely to die or suffer serious injuries from those outdoor sports than those who come to such sports later in life.

I don't buy it.

In fact, my personal experience suggests that just the opposite is true: Kids who participate in outdoor sports as youngsters learn caution and safety consciousness early in their lives, and those qualities serve them well during their fearless teens and invincible 20s.

Alaskan mountaineer and bush pilot Paul Claus, owner and operator of Ultima Thule Outfitters in Wrangell-St. Elias National Park, once told me that most deaths of bush pilots in Alaska occur before the pilots have been flying for five years.

For more on safety in the outdoors, please see Chapter 9: Keeping Your Kids Safe, page 81.

Pilots who make it through those first critical years, Paul explained, by definition have survived enough close calls to have become extra cautious, to know when to refuse to fly or turn back or set a plane down despite the demands of a pushy client.

The same sort of learning curve holds true for outdoor sports, extreme or otherwise. Time and again, I've read accounts of young mountaineers dying or almost dying because they kept climbing when, had they been more experienced, they'd have known to turn back.

By contrast, the advantage of introducing your children to adrenaline-charged outdoor sports as pre-teens is that, during those all-important early years, you'll be on hand to urge caution and instill common sense in them. That way, by the time your children reach their teens and 20s, those values will be built into their psyches. Your children will call upon their reservoirs of caution and common sense when other, less experienced friends try to convince them to ride an avalanche chute on their snowboards or run a rapid that is beyond their abilities in their kayaks.

How, then, to instill common sense in your children? Easy: Set a good example.

Always wear a helmet. Double and triple check your knots. Scout any suspect rapids. Be cautious, and your child will naturally learn by your example to be cautious, too.

One great thing about being openly conservative when participating in outdoor sports with your kids is that the more conservative you are, the more exciting and adrenaline-charged the endeavor will appear to your children.

Take top-rope rock climbing, in which the rope runs from your belay stance up to its anchor point at the top of the cliff and back down to where it is knotted into the climbing harness. As long as your rope is well placed and protected, top roping is the safest form of climbing there is. You simply take in the slack in the rope as your children climb, then lower your children to the ground when they tire or reach the top. Simple and safe.

Despite that high level of safety, every time I top rope with Taylor and Logan, I double and triple check the anchor point, the configuration of the harness, and the knot that attaches them to the rope. Then I have them climb a few feet and take a fall to be sure the rope catches them correctly before they climb higher. As a result, Taylor and Logan view the outdoor rock climbing they do with me and their friends as a grand and dangerous adventure, and I have no doubt they will continue to treat outdoor climbing with caution and respect as they grow older.

The same holds true for kayaking. Unlike our two boys, Sue and I aren't hard-shell kayakers. Instead, we follow our boys down rivers in inflatable kayaks, which involve different, less demanding paddling skills than those required for hard-shell kayaks. That means it's been up to Taylor and Logan to gauge their ability levels on their own against the increasingly more challenging—and dangerous—rapids they want to run in their hard-shells. Because they started kayaking at age 6 and learned the power and potential danger of moving water at a young age, Taylor and Logan have been in no rush to attempt rapids beyond their ability levels. Best of all, the caution they so comfortably display from the cockpit of a kayak will transfer to other aspects of their lives—if one of them must ever decide as a teenager, for example, whether to climb into the passenger seat of a car being driven by a friend who has been drinking.

Your Own Life Will Be Enriched

I grew up a few blocks from the Animas River. Other than floating it in an inner tube a few times each summer, I hardly knew the river flowing through my hometown existed.

These days, however, I seem to be doing something on or along the river almost daily during the warm months of the year. I know the river's flow levels intimately. I know what specific rapids and holes are like when the river is flowing at 300 cubic feet per second versus 3000, and every level in between. I know the best times of day to run or fish various segments of the river depending on windiness and cloud cover. I know when the rainbow trout in the Gold Medal waters through town are hitting on dry flies on the surface, and when they're only going for underwater nymphs.

I know all this—and love knowing it—because I had kids and

have joined them in learning water sports that are new to me.

Though Sue and I did some flatwater canoeing and sea kayaking before Taylor and Logan were born, swiftly running water was something we didn't know much about. Now we do.

Had we not had children, I have no doubt Sue and I would have continued pursuing flatwater sports and left the whitewater to others. Instead, we love the excitement of the kayaking we do with our boys, and we love the close connection to the natural world that comes from our support of our boys' foray into fly-fishing.

Just as Sue and I have been enriched by participating with our boys in outdoor sports that are new to us, so, too, will you—in terrific ways—when you allow yourself to get turned on by your children to outdoor pursuits that are new to you.

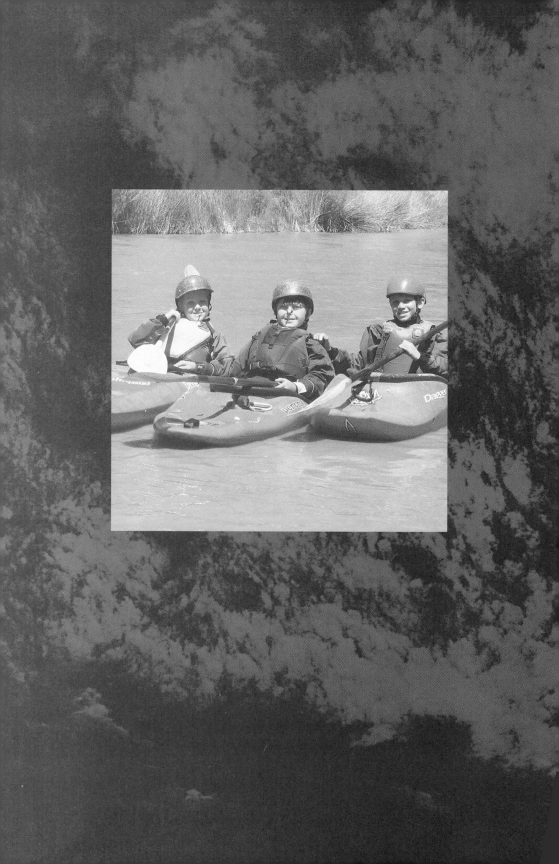

4 Why You Should Do It II: The Philosophical Reasons

The practical reasons for taking on an outdoor action sport or two or three with your kids, as discussed in the last chapter, make logical sense. But to my mind, the philosophical reasons for doing so are far more compelling.

You'll Make Lifelong Connections with Your Kids

Through the simple act of participating in outdoor action sports with your children, you'll connect with them in ways more intense, personal, and life-affirming than you may ever have thought possible, and those shared experiences will form a base of respect and trust upon which solid parent-child relationships are built.

"There are parents who literally say to us, 'This is the first time in a long time I remember having a really good conversation with my child,'" says Ashley Korenblat, owner of Western Spirit Cycling Adventures, which offers family mountain biking trips.

The connections parents forge with their children in the outdoors even tend to stand the trials of teenagerhood. When preadolescent children and parents have tested themselves together in demanding ways in the outdoors, the challenges they face together during the kids' independence-seeking adolescent years become, by comparison, less daunting and more easily managed.

"We've got families who started coming on our trips with their kids before we ever had official 'family' trips," Korenblat says. "They've come every year or every other year, straight through their kids' teen years, and the kids have loved doing our trips with their parents the whole time. The 'children' in some of our families are in their 20s now, and they still love coming on our trips with their parents."

One of the reasons the bonds between parents and children grow so strong in the outdoors is because of the unique challenges presented by outdoor action sports, especially in the backcountry.

> **The connections parents forge with their children in the outdoors tend to withstand even the trials of teenagerhood.**

"There's a camaraderie that develops during our backcountry trips that definitely transcends peoples' ages," Korenblat says. "If there's a storm, everyone has to deal with it. That makes for a real bonding experience."

High Angle Adventures' Jon Ross says the ultimate bonding experience he has seen comes when parents climb while being belayed by their children.

"The parents tell me how intensely personal it is for them to look down from up there and realize their lives literally are in their kids' hands," Ross says.

Your Kids' Confidence Levels Will Skyrocket

We all want our children to grow up to be confident, independent, and self-reliant individuals, right? There's no better way for kids to develop those qualities than by participating in the challenging, highly individual world of outdoor action sports.

Bruce Leffels, of Charlemont, Massachusetts, is a testament to the confidence boost outdoor sports give kids. Leffels was the child of a single parent. As a kid, he was invited along with the family of a school friend on a number of canoe trips throughout New England. Through his participation in those trips, Leffels developed the confidence to commit himself to paddle sports. As an adult, he and his wife, Karen Blom, founded Zoar Outdoor, a rafting and mountain biking outfitter and whitewater paddling school in Charlemont. Today Zoar trains hundreds of people each year to raft, canoe, and kayak.

Blom says she sees the same increase in confidence levels among the children who participate in Zoar's programs that her husband experienced as a youth. Blom says that many of the kids who become involved with Zoar through the company's after-school programs are timid at the outset.

Five Philosophical Reasons for Outdoor Adventuring with Your Kids

1. You'll make lifelong connections with your kids.

2. Your kids' confidence levels will skyrocket.

3. Your kids will gain a tremendous sense of accomplishment.

4. You'll get to enjoy watching your kids develop a great appreciation for the natural world.

5. Your kids' creative abilities will be enhanced.

"But the more they learn, the more comfortable they become with themselves," she says. "Before long, they consider themselves real kayakers, and that's a big deal for them. Then they end up working for us in the summers, and quite a few have gone on to become instructors for us."

River runner and parent Suzanne Strazza, of Mancos, Colorado, says her two boys exhibit this confidence in the most unexpected ways off the river. Strazza's oldest, 5-year-old Everett, refused to wear his favorite socks, made of bright purple fleece, to kindergarten one day because some of his classmates had razzed him about them the last time he'd worn them. Strazza reminded Everett that the socks were ones he always wore on river trips.

"That perked him right up," she says. "He told me, 'Mom, those guys have probably never been on a river trip. That makes me feel bad for them.'"

Then, reports Strazza, off to school Everett went, purple socks sticking out from the toes of his Tevas.

Your Kids Will Gain a Sense of Accomplishment

Outdoor sports offer endless opportunities for kids to set and attain goals, whether those goals involve climbing peaks, catching waves, or riding stretches of single track on a mountain bike. With such success comes a sense of accomplishment so powerful it almost bursts from children.

Mountain Adventure Seminars owner Kimi Johnson sees it often with the kids she teaches in California. "What's really cool about rock climbing is you don't have to be what most people consider 'normally athletic' to be good at it," Johnson says. "It's more the gawky, awkward kids who are 10 feet tall and weigh 50 pounds who do really well at climbing. Long, gangly kids who are 11 or 12 years old have strength-to-weight ratios that are just off the chart. They come out with us and totally surprise themselves and their classmates, who say things like, 'Wow, check out Jimmy. He couldn't catch a ball to save his life, but he just flew up that route.'"

High Angle Adventures' Jon Ross says individually oriented outdoor sports like climbing can be especially beneficial to kids who may not be as comfortable socially as other children. Ross has worked with dyslexic children, for example, and he has seen the benefits that accrue for kids who might generally be picked last for team sports or who are considered "losers" by their classmates.

"In climbing," says Ross, "you've got a kid who's never stepped off the ground, and within 10 or 15 minutes—we're not talking four years of high school—this kid has gone from failure to success."

That, Ross says, "is an enormously powerful thing."

And it's true of all outdoor action sports.

You'll Get to Enjoy Watching Your Kids Develop a Great Appreciation for the Natural World

A few years ago, while waiting for the Fourth of July fireworks to begin near the small mountain town of Silverton, Colorado, Taylor and Logan and the two children of our friends Mark and Jeanne Pastore came up with a plan: They would collect shiny rocks and sell them to passersby. In short order, the four little entrepreneurs earned a little more than $10.

Mark, Jeanne, Sue, and I expected the kids to divvy up their money and spend it on ice-cream cones. Instead, after conferring among themselves, they told us they wanted to donate the money to the Dolores River Coalition, a local effort to convince government officials to re-water the Dolores River below McPhee Dam in western Colorado. (Once a thriving fishery and home to endangered river otters, the river has been reduced to a trickle after the installation of a dam a decade ago.)

I'll confess that the four kids long had heard complaints from Jeanne and Mark and Sue and me about the death of the Dolores. No doubt, their decision to donate the proceeds of their rock sales was a response to our oft-stated discontent. Even so, I don't believe the kids would have thought to donate the money to the Dolores fund merely in answer to our concerns. I have no doubt the kids' idea was born of their awareness of man's impact on the natural world—an awareness gained as a result of having spent large chunks of their young lives floating on and camping alongside waterways and, in so doing, learning to appreciate rivers and deplore their destruction.

In my sons and in other children with whom I've spent time outdoors, I see a natural tendency toward caring for and protecting the natural world. These tendencies manifest in ways that far transcend simply donating money to a cause. I see it in those kids' desire to follow leave-no-trace ethics around campsites, in their efforts to save bugs rather than crush them underfoot, and in their natural inclination to pick up trash along a riverbank or trail.

It Enhances Your Kids' Creativity and Innovativeness

Outdoor sports are individual endeavors that demand individual responses. Every attempt at a bouldering move, every run skied, every wave surfed is unique.

Jack Turner, who produces the television show *Next Snow Search*, a snow-sport X Games for kids, says it's that individuality—that opportunity for endless creativity and innovation—that sets outdoor sports apart from team sports and other modern "thrills" of choice, like video games and theme parks.

"A video game requires no creativity whatsoever," Turner says. "You can get better at it, but what you're getting better at is a computer program designed by someone else."

Theme parks are even worse, he says. "A roller coaster takes the exact same route every single time," says Turner. "It may scare you, but it's all fake. A sack of rocks can ride a roller coaster."

Outdoor sports that involve camping are especially beneficial to kids' creativity. One of the best things about camping out is that time slows down. Cut off from television and video games and released from their busy everyday schedules, kids have time while camping to actually get bored—and to learn there's a lot of creative fun to be had on the far side of boredom.

The most fun I've seen Taylor and Logan have on some of our trips has been after they first grew tired of hanging out around camp. Only then were they called upon to be truly creative. Only then did they invent their own kingdoms in the trees and rocks and on the beaches surrounding camp. Only then did they lead imaginary expeditions, wage centuries-long battles against the forces of evil, and build intricate stick villages and beach waterways that could be flooded and rebuilt over and over again. I've never seen my boys more truly and fully creative, more truly and fully alive, than during those instances—all without the need for crayons and paints and pencils and paper.

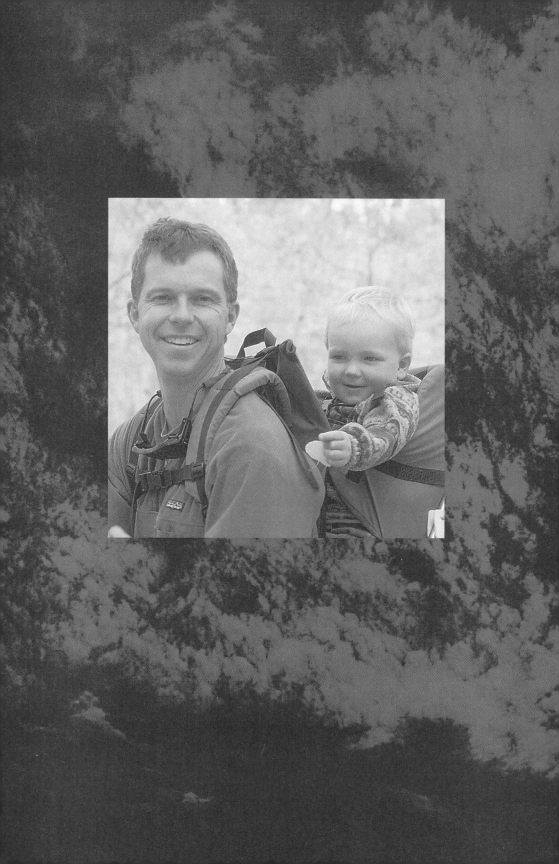

Getting Started:
5 When Your Kids Are Teeny Tiny Tots

S ue and I began "dayhiking" with Taylor when he was a toddler. Those hikes generally entailed car camping and wandering around with Taylor near our campsites. When he grew tired, we'd load him in our child-carrier backpack and set off for longer walks.

One such excursion took us down a slickrock drainage in southeastern Utah's canyon country. Taylor rode contentedly on my back, having worn himself out playing on shelves of sandstone near our camp before we set off.

There were a few clouds in the afternoon sky, but not enough to explain the drops that hit my bare calves every couple of minutes as we hiked along the canyon bottom, aiming for a 100-foot dryfall and the great downcanyon view our guidebook promised would greet us there. I suspected one of Taylor's juice bottles, stored in the bottom pocket of the pack, had a loose lid. I stopped while Sue checked to see if my supposition was correct.

"It's not one of the juice bottles," she said flatly.

It took me a moment to catch on. "Ooohhh," I said finally. "We'd better get him changed."

She rummaged in the pack some more.

"Um. We left the extra diapers at camp."

I looked over my shoulder at her. "Guess it's time to head back."

The drips became steadier during our return. Then, still a good distance from the trailhead, Taylor let loose, drenching my back and legs and providing a deluged end to our shortened hike.

Several years after our wet dayhike with Taylor, Sue and I and Taylor, then 7, and Logan, then 5, set off from home for a fall backpacking trip in Utah's Canyonlands National Park with another family with kids.

An early-season cold front swept toward us during our drive to the park. By the time we reached the turnoff to Canyonlands, light snow was sifting from a gray sky. Continuing on to the park and setting off despite the bad weather made no sense; the kids would have no fun hiking into the teeth of the storm.

After conferring at the side of the highway, we aimed our two-car caravan up the road to Moab and got motel rooms for the night. We managed a short afternoon hike near town despite the biting wind and spitting snow, then enjoyed dinner out followed by an evening of swimming-pool and hot-tub play.

The fast-moving front cleared out overnight, so we headed back down the highway to Canyonlands in the morning and managed to take our fall desert backpacking trip after all— albeit for only one night instead of two. As things turned out, our backpacking trip wasn't a complete success as planned, but it was a success nonetheless, and the evening of pool play at the motel was perfectly enjoyable, too.

Measuring Success Differently

The first few times you try outdoor sports with your youngsters, don't expect total success—in the traditional sense of the word, anyway. You'll likely spend far more time preparing for whatever sport you've chosen to undertake than you will actually undertaking it. Much will go wrong—small hands will get cold, necks will get sunburned, throats will become parched. Boots won't fit, helmet straps will come unfastened, bike chains will wrap themselves around derailleurs. And, of course, it'll rain.

But you have to begin somewhere. Remember, things will get better, but only after you learn to measure success differently than you do as an adult.

Your first attempts at taking to the outdoors adventurously with your kids may be better or worse than our dripping-diaper hike with Taylor, or our shortened backpacking trip in Canyonlands. Regardless, the outcomes of your first attempts most likely won't match your rosy projections for them, no matter how hard you try to keep those projections in check. There simply are too many variables that come into play—weather, gear, sniffly noses, full diapers, projectile vomiting—when tackling outdoor sports with youngsters. That fact remains true no matter how tame, from an adult standpoint, those activities may be.

Moreover, for you as a parent, taking on outdoor action sports with kids entails a significant amount of work. Outdoor sports require lots of gear. Even simple activities such as dayhiking and peak bagging require the right clothing and footwear. Other, more active outdoor sports require far more in the way of equipment: sport-specific helmets, highly specialized clothing and footwear, and various means of conveyance, from telemark skis to surfboards to mountain bikes to kayaks.

Combine those requirements with kids' ever-present need for parental aid, supervision, and encouragement, and you'll understand why the vast majority of parents opt for a trip to Disney World over a climb up Mt. Whitney. As a result, however, they never learn how fantastic—how absolutely worth all the effort—outdoor adventuring with kids really is.

> When you start kids young in outdoor sports, it's much easier if you learn to measure success differently than you do as an adult.

The Benefits of Repetition

During the years when our boys were very young, Sue and I regularly returned with them to the same area of Utah for dayhiking, short backpacking trips, and aimless exploration. We also rafted the same river regularly during those early years, growing comfortable with the campsites and rapids along the way. Returning to the same stretch of water for river running and the same region of

Three Keys to Outdoor Adventuring with Youngsters

Accept Reality: You're the parent of little kids now. The definition of outdoor adventure is far different for them than it may have been for you in the past.

Repeat Yourself: Grow comfortable with your little ones in the outdoors by returning to places and repeating trips that work well for you and your kids.

Remember: It's the Journey. When things go wrong, as they inevitably will, remember that each outing you take with your youngsters is a step along the way. Soon, the trips you'll eventually take with your kids—who will grow up in an instant—will run smoothly and easily. When they do, you'll look back longingly on the more difficult early trips when your kids were bright-eyed, wonder-filled youngsters.

high desert for camping and backpacking proved healthy for all of us during those early years for two reasons:

1. Children crave structure and routine. The repetitious nature of our early outdoor activities with our boys answered that craving.

2. Knowing where we were going made our early trips easier for Sue and me by removing one unknown from the long list of unknowns that accompanied us each time we set out.

Not until the boys were older did we begin to seek new venues for our adventures. At that point, thanks to the base of experience we'd by then built up, both we and the boys were ready for the new locations we explored and the kayaking, mountain biking, rock climbing, longer backpacking trips, and other outdoor sports we pursued.

Avoiding the National Park Family Meltdown

Ashley Korenblat of Western Spirit Cycling offers a vivid description of what she and other Western Spirit guides have come to call the "national park family meltdown."

Though the meltdown can and does happen anywhere, Korenblat has witnessed it virtually every time she's taken a Western Spirit group to the rim of the collapsed Mt. Mazama volcano in Oregon's Crater Lake National Park. There, the trail begins for the 1-mile hike from the volcano's rim 700 vertical feet down to the shore of Crater Lake.

"For a lot of families traveling on their own, the hike down to the lake is a big thing," Korenblat says. "The parents have talked about it with their kids. Everybody's excited about it."

Then the families show up at the volcano's rim. From across the parking lot, where she's readying her own group for the hike, Korenblat watches as trouble brews.

The parents look down at the lake from the trailhead and realize they've over-promised: The hike is much tougher than they had anticipated. Many call off the hike right there in the parking lot, leading to a meltdown as the kids, primed for the biggest adventure of their family's vacation, come unglued.

Other parents forge ahead.

"The kids are so excited that the parents can't bring themselves to say no," says Korenblat. "So off they go, even if something inside them is telling them maybe they shouldn't."

Of course, going down is easy. And staying too long at the lake is even easier. But in the end, the families must hike back up the trail. Many have run out of water by then. The all-important snacks children need to keep moving along a trail—especially a steep uphill trail like the one leading back to the rim of Mt. Mazama from Crater Lake—have long since been eaten.

Things turn ugly. The afternoon sun blazes down. The kids and parents get thirstier and hungrier and crankier. The minutes tick by. The hiking parties slow, then slow some more.

"By the time they get back to the parking lot, they're all fit to be tied," Korenblat says. "So much for the big family adventure."

The key to avoiding the national park family meltdown, whether you're in a national park or not, is to keep your goals in check.

A mile hike down to Crater Lake and back may not seem like much to you, but with kids, things change. A mile hike can be a full-on adventure for children of the right age, and for you as a parent as well, or it may turn into a forced march.

That's why, when tackling outdoor sports with your youngsters, it's crucial to start small. Understand that a

How to Enjoy Outdoor "Adventuring" with Your Youngsters

- Slow down.
- Leave the how-many-miles-did-you-run/hike/bike/paddle mentality at home.
- Learn to appreciate what it is your kids so naturally appreciate about the outdoors, because what they appreciate is great stuff.
- Realize that the early exploratory years with your kids will be over all too soon.

simple outdoor activity that is within your children's abilities may not be your idea of adventure, but it will be to your kids, as long as you allow it to be. By choosing simple adventures at which your children succeed, you'll get to savor along with them the excitement that will result from those adventures—excitement that will be over and gone before you know it.

Appreciating What Your Kids Appreciate

"Dad! Look!" Taylor, then 5, called as he ran toward me, his cupped hand outstretched. "I found a piece of Indian pottery!"

I waited without great anticipation.

Taylor and I were taking a break from a hike in Mule Canyon, a low-walled cut in southeastern Utah's Cedar Mesa, while Sue and Logan played back at camp. Before he'd come running to me, Taylor had been floating reed rafts in a trickle of water tumbling over ledges of slickrock in the shade of a cottonwood. We were only two flat, easy-hiking miles from the trailhead. Two miles.

For 10 years before we had kids, Sue and I had explored the sinuous canyons of southeastern Utah the best way we knew how, by putting boot sole to slickrock. We'd backpacked established trails end to end, bushwhacked unnamed drainages, climbed cliff walls to reach hidden nooks and out-of-the-way alcoves.

In that time, we'd encountered thousands of potsherds—broken pieces of pottery left behind by the ancient Indians of the region known as the Anasazi. In every case, however, the potsherds we'd found had been displayed for us, arrayed like museum artifacts on flat pieces of stone beneath overhangs by hikers who had preceded our arrival. Never had either of us found a potsherd on our own.

"Look," Taylor insisted. He dropped what was sure to be a piece of gray shale into my palm and gazed at me with glowing expectation.

I feigned excitement before looking down at his 2-inch-by-2-inch discovery, hoping he hadn't noticed the doubt in my eyes.

Taylor's find curved inward in manmade fashion. The side facing me was unnaturally smooth. I shivered and turned it over in my hand. The outward-curving side was corrugated with row upon row of shark-tooth-like indentations.

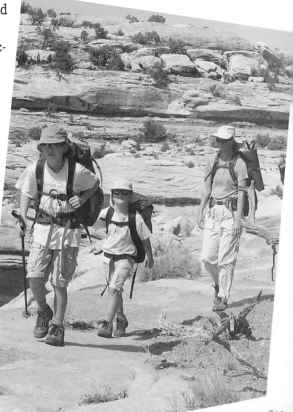

I laughed out loud and tousled Taylor's hair.

"You're right," I said. "It's Anasazi."

"Yesssss!" he cried happily, his blue eyes sparkling.

I grinned back at him, chastened by my doubts and thrilled for Taylor and his fully justified excitement about his treasure.

I found out that day how best to enjoy adventuring in the outdoors with youngsters: The key, Taylor taught me, is to slow down. Leave the how-many-miles-did-you-run/hike/bike/paddle mentality at home. Learn to appreciate what it is your kids so naturally appreciate about the outdoors, because what they appreciate is great stuff when, as I learned, you take the time to recognize it.

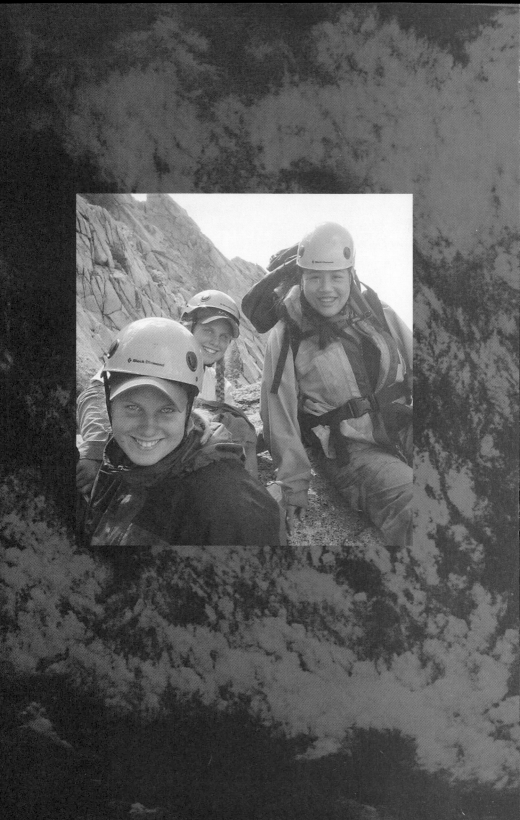

6 Getting Started II: When Your Kids Are Older

One way to get started on a life of outdoor adventure with your kids is to go at it full bore like the Jackson family.

Ever since their children were youngsters, pro kayaker and father Eric Jackson and mother Kristine Jackson have spent much of each year with daughter Emily and son Dane living in a recreational vehicle. They travel from kayak event to kayak event in their RV with countless stops along the way for noncompetitive river play.

"I always said I wanted my kids to live extraordinary lives," says Kristine. "When Eric and I came upon the idea of hitting the road, we just jumped on it."

Emily and Dane, members of the US Junior Freestyle Kayak Team, spend up to 200 days a year paddling various rivers with their father, a former world champion and a member of the men's freestyle team. Kristine, who doesn't kayak, homeschools the kids in the family RV.

"We could stay home and watch TV," Kristine says, "but that wouldn't really be living."

Kids' Abilities

Most of us aren't able to travel the world full time in search of outdoor adventure with our kids. But there's a great lesson in the Jackson family's experience: They have proven that children take to outdoor adventure with ease, and that it's simply up to us, as parents, to present it to them.

49

Dane Jackson's story provides a perfect example. In 2004, at age 11, Dane first made the US Junior Freestyle Kayak Team, which consists of the country's three best freestyle paddlers ages 18 and under.

Yes, you read that right. *Eleven*.

Tips for Getting Started When Your Kids Are Older

- Be prepared for and ready to accept the grumbling that often comes from older kids who are faced with something new, even if it's the opportunity to try an awesome new outdoor sport (likely at significant expense to you). More than likely, the grumbling will disappear as soon as your kids get into the sport. If it doesn't, there are lots of other great outdoor sports to try.

- Remember, no law says you have to get started in a new sport hand in hand with your children, especially when they're older (say, those ages 10 and up) and therefore beginning to explore and appreciate their independence. Instead, you may need to give older kids the space and opportunity to try a new sport for a bit on their own. Once they're accomplished at a given sport, you can then give it a try—with them acting in a leadership role and helping you out.

- Understand that, like Dane Jackson making the three-man US Junior Freestyle Kayak Team at age 11, your kids quickly will become capable of incredible feats at whatever outdoor sports you take up with them. There's no use blowing out a knee or shoulder trying to catch up or keep up with them. Better to take pride in your kids' accomplishments while comfortably tagging along behind.

"When you pull a kayak trick, there's a lot you have to do at once," Kristine says. "No one was entirely sure a kid as young as Dane could put it all together. But we found out younger kids like him really can do it."

The point here is not to glorify the benefits of competitive success for youngsters participating in outdoor action sports. There's no doubt Dane is good at what he does because he's spent his entire young life doing it. Still, that doesn't take away from the fact that he is, indeed, capable of doing incredible things in a kayak. And that's the point: Kids can do amazing things in the outdoors at very young ages, provided they're given the chance.

Since the family company, Jackson Kayak, introduced the Fun 1 kayak for little-kid paddlers, Kristine says she and Eric have been inundated with videos of kids doing wild moves in big water in their kid-size boats.

"Before we came out with the Fun 1, a lot of people said, 'Well, it's just Dane,'" says Kristine. "But we've gotten videos of 7-year-olds running Class III rapids and 8-year-olds doing big-drop waterfalls. It's apparent it's not just Dane; lots of kids can do this if they have the right equipment."

When it comes to learning new activities, the brains of preadolescents are sponges. For absolute proof, all I've had to do is watch my boys try sport after sport and get a good grip on each within minutes of trying it.

Given that reality, the best way to introduce your kids to the wide world of outdoor sports is to turn them loose. Introduce them to sports that interest you, but also let them try whatever catches their fancy.

In particular, exploring sports with your kids that are new to you as well as to your children presents terrific opportunities for you to spend time with them on the same level. From a connecting-with-your-kids standpoint, all such activities—attempting to rig a raft, learning to

51

secure a harness while taking a rock climbing course together, or teaming up to figure out how clipless mountain bike pedals work—are as tremendously valuable as they are all too rare in most parent-child relationships these days.

Don't shy away from introducing your kids to several outdoor sports, either. All outdoor sports compliment one another in some way because all either harness or confront the force of gravity.

The Magic Number Six

Until your kids are 5 or so, you'll be outdoor "adventuring" with them in ways that are exciting and fun to them, but wouldn't be to you as an adult if you weren't with your kids. If you dayhike or backpack with your youngsters, your trips will be short. If you run rivers, your kids will be passengers. If you bike, your kids will be behind you in a trailer or trail-a-bike.

Along about age 6 or so, things change. As if by magic, your kids will be ready to take on the world of outdoor adventure on their own. At that point, it simply will be up to you to:

1. Give them the opportunity.
2. Keep them safe.
3. And hold on for the ride of your life.

SLICKROCK LEARNING CURVE

Sue and I first mountain biked the now world-famous Slickrock Trail outside Moab, Utah, in the mid-1980s. At the time, the trail was used more by its original denizens, motorcyclists, than by neophyte mountain bikers like Sue and me. The trailhead, now a huge paved parking lot with bathrooms and dumpsters, was merely a wide spot alongside the dirt road leading from town.

Riding the trail with our clunky, first-generation mountain bikes wasn't easy, but it was incredibly fun. We returned to ride the trail several times in the years that followed.

Then came Taylor and Logan.

While the boys were baby and toddler age, we car camped, dayhiked, rafted, and explored backcountry areas in gradually widening circles with our boys. But we didn't return to the Slickrock Trail. Nor did we do any of the high-altitude mountaineering that had been such a big part of our lives before kids. We stopped free-heel skiing the steeps and deeps and instead stuck to telemarking on flats and gentle slopes, the boys in packs on our backs.

Don't get me wrong, I'm not complaining. Sue and I loved every minute of those early years with our boys, and we miss them terribly now that they're behind us. But behind us they are.

Don't shy away from introducing your kids to several outdoor sports.

Eventually, Taylor, followed quickly by Logan, learned to ski, ride a two-wheeler, paddle a kayak, hike longer distances, and climb higher heights. In the span of a few short months, Sue and I went from the short walks and lizard chasing our boys enjoyed during their early years to the adrenaline-charged sports we'd always enjoyed in the outdoors on our own, except this time with our boys participating right alongside us.

Nowhere was the change more apparent than at the Slickrock Trail. After many years away, we showed up at the Slickrock Trailhead one November day when Taylor was 6. The weather was cool and blustery, but the parking lot was crowded with 20- and 30-something riders hot for the trail. Not sure what we were in for, we set Taylor up with his miniature mountain bike and walked along the trail leading Logan, then 4, by the hand while Taylor rode.

As we had hoped, the redrock turned out to be as terrific a biking playground for Taylor as it always had been for Sue and me. We took turns spotting Taylor as he attempted steep climbs and tight turns. We stood back and watched nervously as he swooped downhill and pedaled gentler uphill stretches. After an hour or so, when Sue,

Logan, and I were beyond bored, we had to force Taylor to head back with us to the parking lot.

Since that day, we've returned to ride the Slickrock Trail regularly as a family. Logan did his first mini-rides on the trail at age 5, while Taylor completed his first loop of the entire 11-mile trail at age 9, the same age as plenty of other kids we know.

The story here is similar to that of Dane Jackson. It isn't that Sue and I have amazingly talented bike-riding kids. Rather it's that, from age 6 on, our boys have been fully capable of doing stuff in the outdoors that is totally fun for us to do right along with them.

Guided Family Adventures

Taking to the outdoors with Taylor and Logan on a do-it-ourselves basis has been fairly easy for Sue and me because we did a lot in the outdoors before our boys were born. The same no doubt is true of the success pro-kayaker Eric Jackson has had introducing his children to white-water kayaking.

If, conversely, you didn't spend a great deal of time in the outdoors before you had kids, and you now want to share the outdoors with them in adventurous ways, your best bet may be to get started by signing up for a guided activity.

The decisions made by outfitters on behalf of the families they guide are based on years of experience at learning what works best.

Guides and instructors with experience leading families are available for any outdoor sport you wish to tackle. You can begin your search for an appropriate guide or school by flipping through the latest editions of *Outside* and *National Geographic Adventure* magazines. Both publications include family-focused articles and outfitter advertisements, in keeping with their parent-aged readers.

If you know a specific sport you'd like to try, check out any magazines that cover the sport you have in mind, as well as those magazines' websites. Use the internet to check the sites of outfitters and schools, and then ask for references (and be sure to call them!) before plunking down your money. All outfitters can scare up a few good reviews for their websites; the only way to get a real feel for whether an outfitter will make a good fit for your family is to talk personally with parents who have already used the outfitter or school.

Western Spirit Cycling's Ashley Korenblat notes that one of the best attributes of outfitted trips is that they virtually guarantee families will not suffer from any version of a "national park family meltdown." Because the family trips offered by outfitters are tried, tested, and constantly refined and improved, the decisions made by outfitters on behalf of the families they guide are the right ones.

"When you go with an outfitter," Korenblat says, "you know you'll be part of an itinerary that's within the ability level of everyone. You can count on a trip that will be enjoyable rather than frustrating—or maybe even down-right dangerous."

One such outfitter with programs that lend themselves to beginner families is Charlemont, Massachusetts-based Zoar Outdoor, located on the banks of the Deerfield River in the Berkshire Mountains two-and-a-half hours from Boston. Zoar has created canoeing and kayaking courses specifically for families in recent years.

"At this point, families are 30 percent of our business," says Zoar owner Karen Blom. "Families have been a grow-ing segment for us, and we've added courses in response."

For several years, Zoar has offered two-day parent/child novice whitewater kayaking and canoeing clinics. In 2004, Zoar began offering what it billed as its Family Fun Week, a full week of kayaking instruction designed to take an entire family from novice to intermediate in a few days. Zoar also offers a Family Sampler Week that enables fami-lies to try out several active outdoor sports—rock climb-ing, mountain biking, rafting, kayaking, and canoeing—with the help of guides in a single week.

Guided trips and instructor-led courses are a great way to get started, especially for families who haven't spent much time in the outdoors. "Many of our families come to us from Boston or New York because we're close by and they don't have to go all the way up into the wilds of Maine to find out if these sports are something they're interested in," Blom says. "For them, a simple rafting trip on Class II water is a huge experience."

Between Do-It-Yourself and Guided Trips

One middle-ground approach to getting started on a new outdoor sport with your kids is demonstrated by John and Mary Mummery, the parents of four kids who enjoy scuba diving, camping, climbing, and other outdoor pursuits.

A few years ago, the Mummerys decided to undertake a family backcountry canoe trip in northern Minnesota's Boundary Waters Canoe Area Wilderness. John and Mary were well-versed in backpacking and whitewater rafting, but they'd never undertaken a paddle-and-portage canoe trip like the Boundary Waters adventure they were planning with their kids.

Faced with the same situation, I suspect I would have tried to convince Sue to simply rent canoes, shove off with our boys, and slowly figure things out as we went. I'm sure we would have survived such a trip, but I'm also sure the trip would have been less than optimally fun given the steep learning curve we'd have faced.

The Mummerys are far smarter than I am. They had no desire to join a guided Boundary Waters trip, but they also recognized that they could learn a lot from a guide. So instead of investing in an outfitter-organized trip, they hired a guide for half a day in Minnesota before they set off on their own.

The half day was spent on the shore and surface of a roadside lake. There, the guide ran through the gear the Mummerys needed for their trip. He showed them how to pack a canoe for a Boundary Waters trip, how to paddle and maneuver a loaded canoe, and how best to accomplish a portage. He also provided the Mummerys with safety advice and campsite-selection tips.

"The knowledge the guide shared with us was worth every minute it took to learn and every penny it cost us," John says.

The Mummerys headed into the Boundary Waters wilderness with their kids the next morning. Armed with the right knowledge, they pulled off their five-day trip without a hitch.

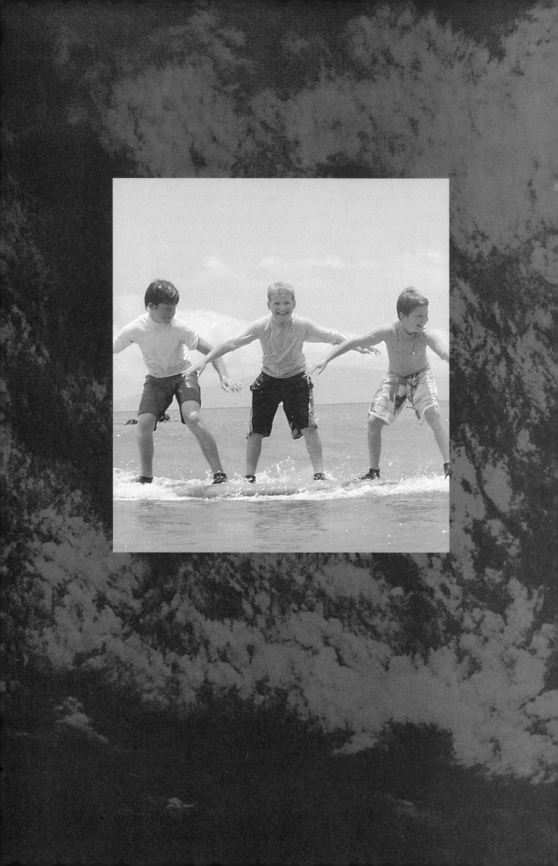

7 What Does Extreme Really Mean?

I tasted death for the first time on a hot summer day when I was 12. My older brother and I were navigating the Animas River through Durango on a pair of inflated truck inner tubes. Wearing what was considered appropriate safety gear for the time—thin foam water-ski belts around our waists—we drifting lazily through Durango in cutoff jeans and Converse All-Stars, our bare chests to the noonday sun.

Near the end of our trip, we headed down Smelter Rapid, the only whitewater of any consequence in town. Today, Smelter has been narrowed and excavated to create a tight, Class III drop. Back then, the rapid consisted of the river simply cascading over a series of car-size boulders. Kevin bobbed between the rocks without incident, but I happened to float over one of the rocks, drop off its downstream side, and flip off my tube. The curling water below the rock sucked me beneath the surface, in spite of the "flotation" device around my waist. In an instant I was trapped, suspended a couple of feet below the surface.

What I recall most from my entrapment is the strange sense of curiosity that took hold of me. As the water spun me like clothing in a dryer, I looked about with detached wonder. My perspective switched from seeing the dim light of the sky above to the dark bottom of the hole and back to the light, over and over again.

There was time enough for me to consider the oddity of my situation—a 12-year-old kid twisting lazily underwater, light and sky and air suddenly far away. Then, just as I began to sense the need to breathe, and so just as the first seed of fear sowed itself deep in my gut, the curling water spit me out.

I surfaced to a yell of relief from Kevin and dog-paddled to where he waited downstream with my tube.

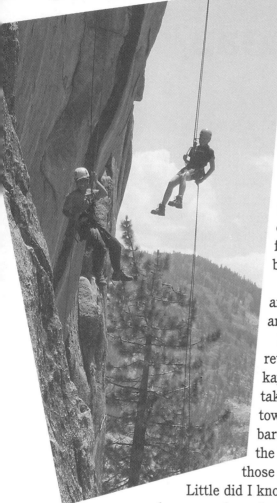

Defining Extreme

Six years after my underwater experience in Smelter, I left Durango for college. When I moved back to town with Sue 15 years later, when Taylor was 2 and Logan a newborn, I eyed manicured Smelter Rapid with respect—and growing interest. What opportunities for extreme adventure did the river hold for Sue and me and our two little boys?

It took me a few years to learn the answer to that question. And the answer wasn't at all what I expected.

In looking at the Animas upon my return to Durango, I saw only the many kayakers in their colorful boats who had taken to playing in the river through town in the years since my childhood. I barely noticed the fly-fishermen who, like the kayakers, had taken to the river in those intervening years as well.

Little did I know that the sport of fly-fishing would play as much a role in defining "extreme" to me as the sport of kayaking. Not until years later would I come to know, through the bringing up of my sons along the banks of the Animas, that extreme isn't necessarily the stuff of extreme sport videos. Extreme is defined by the individual, not the sport. It's what is in each of us and each of our kids.

It appeared clear to me, as I stood watching Smelter Rapid upon my return to Durango, that the many kayakers running the new-and-improved rapid were having loads of fun. No doubt, Taylor and Logan would want to experience Smelter themselves when they grew older, just as I had wanted to as a kid. But how to introduce them to whitewater and to kayaking without endangering them as I had endangered myself, especially since Sue and I knew nothing about kayaking ourselves? How to begin exploring the definition of extreme with a couple of little boys and the big river at our disposal?

I turned to whitewater canoe and kayak master Kent Ford for the answer. Ford is a national-level whitewater coach, two-time world champion whitewater paddler, and former manager of North Carolina's Nantahala Outdoor Center, the largest canoeing and kayaking school in the world. These days, he produces whitewater training videos through his company, Performance Video.

I was ready for Ford to give me a list of instructions, starting with "enroll your kids in a class" (though at the time no one in the country offered kayaking classes for kids younger than 8). Instead, Ford told me the best way to start a kid kayaking was simply to "throw a boat in the water and throw your kid in with it." Give them a taste of the water and kayaking first, he said, then move on to instruction.

Though many parents introduce their kids to kayaking only through official courses (a perfectly fine way to go), the approach suggested by Ford appealed to the do-it-ourselves philosophy that Sue and I share. Not long after Taylor turned 6, we picked up a used kayak, paddle, and personal flotation device, or PFD, at a local whitewater gear swap. We headed for a nearby lake, where we did as Ford had suggested. Before long, Taylor was paddling happily back and forth across the water. Next we took him to a calm stretch of the Animas, where he picked up the idea of paddling in a slight current. A few weeks later,

Extreme isn't necessarily the stuff of extreme sport videos.

while Sue, Logan, and I rafted, Taylor ran 56 miles of the mostly flatwater San Juan River alongside us in his kayak.

Over time, Taylor received kayaking instruction and learned rolling, paddling, and safety techniques through friends and as a member of the local whitewater team.

Now Taylor is as comfortable flipping in whitewater and rolling back upright in his boat as he is sitting on a couch eating popcorn. For his part, Logan is fast mastering the sport of kayaking, too.

Redefining Extreme

The same year Sue and I introduced Taylor to kayaking, a pair of fly-fishermen worked their way upstream past where we happened to be camped on the banks of Calf Creek in south-central Utah.

From the moment Taylor saw the two men, he was captivated by the beauty of what they were up to, the graceful back-and-forth motion of the fly-fishing cast, and the gentle landing of the fly on the water. As soon as the fishermen passed from view, Taylor insisted we tie a length of string onto a willow switch for him. He then proceeded to flail the surface of the creek with his makeshift pole for the next hour.

At first glance, the sports of kayaking and fly-fishing seem as different as can be, but they can both be considered extreme in their own way.

Taylor refused to let go of the idea of fly-fishing after we returned home from our trip. When he wouldn't listen to our explanation that he was too young for fly-fishing, we finally allowed him to use his own money to buy an inexpensive rod and reel from a department store.

He started out practicing his cast in our driveway while I read up on how to tie a leader to a fly line, a tippet to a leader, and a fly to a tippet. I asked around for good sites in our area for a little kid to try fly-fishing, and we set out for them. Within short order—despite his parents' beliefs to the contrary—Taylor was catching fish on flies in creeks near our home.

Simply catching fish wasn't enough, however. Before long, Taylor decided he had to learn to tie his own flies as well. This time we paid for his beginner fly-tying kit and his enrollment in a beginner fly-tying class at a local fly-fishing shop. Again, we assumed Taylor's grand plan to master the art of fly-tying would be short-lived. Again, Taylor proved us wrong.

Though the class ran an hour past his bedtime several nights in a row, Taylor diligently worked his way through it, a second-grader among men and women in their 20s and 30s. He then began tying and selling simple flies to the shop at which he'd taken the class.

Today, Sue and I still don't know much about catch-and-release fly-fishing. Taylor, on the other hand, continues to fish like a fiend. And the flies he ties on the professional vise we eventually broke down and purchased for him are increasingly sophisticated—and in high demand among the local fishermen to whom he sells them.

Taylor taught Logan to fly-fish when Logan was 7. The brothers now leapfrog pools along the streams in our area. In addition, Taylor is teaching Logan the art of fly-tying, and the two have plans to start their own fly-tying company someday.

Extreme Sports vs. Extreme Kids

At first glance, the sports of kayaking and fly-fishing seem as different as can be. Kayaking is all about adrenaline and fast-twitch muscles. Fly-fishing is about artistry and careful pursuit, 8-foot wisps of carbon fiber wielded silently above calm

63

pools. Yet both sports depend, at their base level, on flowing water for all the wonders and possibilities they present their participants.

"Wait," I can already hear you saying. "Kayaking's an
'extreme' sport, sure. But what's so extreme
about fly-fishing?"

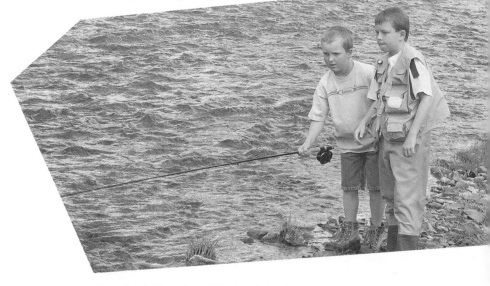

To which I reply: This book isn't necessarily about
"extreme" sports. It's about how to connect with and raise
Extreme Kids—kids who go all out in life, who, given the
opportunity to experience the outdoors in fun ways as
children, will love, appreciate, protect, and spend time in
the outdoors the rest of their lives.

For the most part, that will mean you'll be introducing
your kids to sports they'll view as radical, cool, and, yes,
extreme. For most kids most of the time, that's where the
most fun is.

But it also will mean that, when it comes to figuring out
what to do with your kids in the outdoors, it'll be up to
you to listen to them. Let them try something they take a
fancy to. Maybe they'll burn out on it in a day or two.
Maybe it'll become their lifelong passion.

Besides, is whitewater kayaking really that much more
extreme than fly-fishing?

At first thought, the answer seems easy: Of course it is.

Video clips of gonzo kayakers are part of every extreme sport highlight reel ever produced. As for fly-fishing? Yawn.

Yet as Taylor and Logan take on ever bigger water in their kayaks, the most worried I am for their safety in the outdoors is when they fly-fish.

Kayaking is a group activity. It has its share of dangers, as do all outdoor sports. But within kayaking's group framework lies much safety. When someone gets in trouble, others are around to help out.

By contrast, fly-fishing is most successfully practiced alone. The farther a fisherman gets from others, the more fish the fisherman catches. Yet solitary fly-fishermen regularly die while fishing: They slip and fall in cold, fast-moving water, their waders fill, and they drown.

It doesn't help that the best fly-fishing in much of the country is in clear waters flowing from the base of dams. Those locations, known as tailwater fisheries, provide excellent conditions for fish and fly-fishing. Problem is, tailwaters are notoriously cold and fickle—and lead to an inordinate number of fly-fishing deaths.

At first, Sue and I required Taylor to wear a personal flotation device every time he fished in rivers as opposed to creeks. Now that he's taller, Taylor has switched from wearing the more dangerous chest waders to safer thigh-high waders, and it's Logan we now require to wear a PFD over his handed-down-from-Taylor chest waders. Even so, every time Taylor and Logan head out into big water with their poles, intent not on staying alive but on catching the next big one, I pace the shore or wade along behind them nervously, wearing my own PFD, making sure they're safe.

Which, then, is really more extreme, whitewater kayaking or fly-fishing?

There's no correct answer.

That's the beauty of outdoor sports, be they adrenaline-filled ocean surfing or meditative sea kayaking: No one's keeping score. Extreme is, or isn't, in the eyes of the participant.

The point isn't extreme sports anyway. The point is extreme, out-there, appreciative, fun-loving, happy kids.

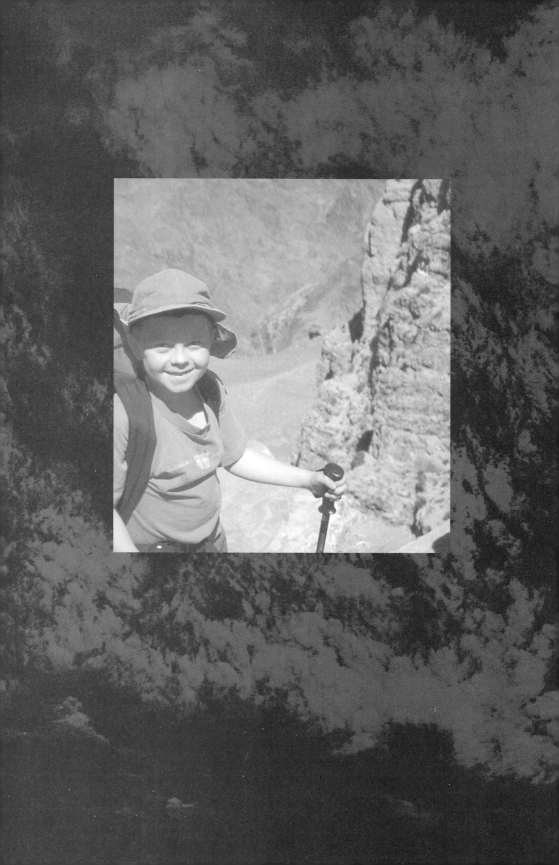

8 The Actual, By-God Doing of the Thing

When Logan was 6 and Taylor 9, Sue and I decided to backpack the Grand Canyon with them. We approached the trip with more than a little trepidation. The trip would entail:

- Seven waterless miles and 5000 vertical feet down the Kaibab Trail to our campsite at Bright Angel Creek.

- After a rest day, 5 miles and 2500 vertical feet up to our next campsite at Indian Gardens.

- Then, after another rest day, another 5 miles and 2500 vertical feet (most of those vertical feet in the steep, switchbacking final 3 miles) out of the canyon on our final day.

- Carrying five days' worth of food and fuel.

- Lugging enough cold-weather gear to survive one of the canyon's occasional spring snowstorms if one happened to hit us during our trip.

- All with a kindergartner and third-grader.

We knew the only way we'd successfully pull off the trip was if we had the boys fully psyched for it. As soon as we learned we'd scored a late March permit for the hike, we began talking it up with them—how demanding it would be, but how certain we were that Taylor and, especially, 6-year-old Logan were capable of it. Up to and throughout the trip, we pitched to the boys the extremism of what

67

they were doing, as well as our confidence that they could pull it off.

The result?

On day one, Logan scurried ahead of us down the Kaibab Trail. He wound up hiking most of the way to the Colorado River with a family from Michigan. During our rest day at the bottom of the canyon, Taylor and Logan gamboled along the banks of Bright Angel Creek while Sue and I limped along behind, our calves aching from the previous day's descent. On day three, the boys tootled up to Indian Gardens with nary a whine.

On day five, in anticipation of the Bright Angel Trail's steep final stretch, Sue and the boys left Indian Gardens at dawn while I remained behind to break down our tent. I caught up with Sue, Taylor, and Logan after 2 miles of hiking. From there, the boys took off ahead of Sue and me. Though we'd loaded Taylor with 15 pounds on his back and Logan with 10, Sue and I didn't see the boys again until we reached the South Rim—30 minutes after they'd topped out.

> **We'd ignored our boys' needs. That is, we'd neglected the all-important pitch.**

We'd promised the boys a fancy breakfast at the refined El Tovar restaurant on the lip of the canyon the day after our trip. I checked my watch when we completed our hike. It was 9:30. El Tovar was still serving breakfast. We walked the half-mile asphalt path to the restaurant, where the maitre d' invited us to leave our packs in a private dining room once favored by Teddy Roosevelt. He then led us to a white-cloth-covered table in the main dining room overlooking the canyon for one of the finest breakfasts we've ever enjoyed.

Four weeks later, Sue and I took advantage of a long April weekend to backpack with the boys into remote Dark Canyon in southeastern Utah. The Sundance Trail that leads to the bottom of Dark Canyon isn't much of a trail at all. Rather, it's a haphazardly cairned route down a steep sandstone talus slope 1500 feet to the canyon bottom.

Sue and I had been biding our time for years, waiting for the boys to grow old enough to backpack Dark Canyon,

called
by
many a
miniature
Grand Canyon
for its desert
beauty and soaring
redrock walls. Now
that the boys had hiked
the Grand, we knew they
were ready for Dark Canyon. They'd done so well in the
Grand Canyon, in fact, that even though the Sundance
Trail promised to be rugged, we felt none of the trepidation we'd felt before setting off down the Kaibab Trail, and
we didn't bother to talk up the trip to the boys.

That turned out to be a big mistake.

The late-spring day we set off was sunny and warm, the
early-summer no-see-ums hadn't yet hatched, and the trail
across the mesa top to the talus slope was smooth and
easy to follow. In other words, everything about the trip
was perfect. Even so, the boys began complaining shortly
after we left the trailhead. Their feet hurt, they said. Their
packs didn't feel right. They were really, really tired.

Sue and I figured out what was going on pretty quickly:
In the case of both our Grand Canyon trip and our Dark
Canyon trip, we'd thought only of ourselves. We'd talked
up the Grand Canyon trip to the boys because of our concern that the trip might be difficult for them, and thus for
us.

After watching the ease with which the boys had hiked
the Grand Canyon, we'd known they could easily handle
Dark Canyon. Because of our own comfort level, we'd

69

ignored our boys' needs. That is, we'd neglected the all-important pitch.

We immediately began offering the boys the same sort of encouragement and positive reinforcement we'd offered them during the Grand Canyon trip. As we neared the

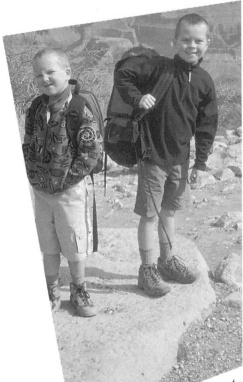

drop into Dark Canyon proper, we talked of how tough downclimbing the steep slope would be, but of how sure we were they could handle it. We spoke in glowing terms of Dark Canyon, of its many comparisons to the Grand Canyon, of how incredible it was that only four weeks after hiking the Grand, the boys were hiking Dark Canyon as well.

Our last-minute sales job worked. It got the boys' minds off the drudgery that is trail hiking to young kids and instead got their minds on what they were about to accomplish.

Taylor and Logan dropped down the talus slope, which was indeed rugged, without complaint. We camped beside Dark Creek and talked up the challenge of reclimbing the slope until we set off to do so two days later, at which point the boys fairly bounded up the steep trail and back to the trailhead.

The Pitch

To all the trips we've taken in the years since, Sue and I have made a point of applying the valuable lesson we learned over the course of our Grand Canyon and Dark Canyon trips: Pitching a trip to your kids isn't about assuring yourself that your kids will be able to make it. (If there's any real concern that they won't be able to complete a trip, you shouldn't be undertaking the trip with them in the first place.) You don't pitch a trip in answer to

your own concerns, we learned. Rather, you pitch an outdoor adventure to your kids to make sure they're excited
about it.

The simple truth is that many aspects of outdoor sports
aren't fun. They're undertaken outdoors, for one thing.
Rain falls outdoors. So does snow. Mosquitoes and horse
flies attack. In addition, certain aspects of outdoor sports

The Importance of the Pitch

Your kids deserve pre-trip and during-trip pitches because
outdoor adventures aren't 100 percent fun for them. From a
kid's perspective, outdoor adventures involve:

■ All the vagaries of the outdoors—rain, snow, cold, wind,
   mosquitoes.

■ Unavoidable periods of little in the way of excitement.

■ Challenging levels of physical endurance.

■ The need for potentially daunting amounts of courage.

are just plain boring for young children. Outdoor adventures may involve long drives to get there, long stretches
of flatwater, lots of walking. At the same time, outdoor
adventures require physical endurance. Often, they're
extremely tiring for kids, and we all know what it's like to
deal with tired children. Moreover, outdoor sports require
real courage. Running a rapid, hiking a cliff-side trail,
catching a 4-foot wave, dropping down a steep incline on a
mountain bike—all can frighten a kid, and that fear can
easily result in a ruined trip.

It's important to look at the outdoor sports you take on
with your kids from *their* perspective. In recognition of
that perspective, it's critical that you *sell* your planned trip
or outing to them. Let them know how fun it's going to be,
but also how intense—and how certain you are that
they're up to the challenge.

When you do that, your kids won't focus on their boredom
or, conversely, their fear. They won't focus on how tired or
uncomfortable they may be. Rather, they'll focus on the
challenge you've set before them and the opportunity

you've given them to meet that challenge. The result? An enjoyable adventure for you and your kids.

Keeping Them Happy

Several years ago, I faced down a potential disaster while floating a flatwater stretch of the Colorado River on the fourth and final day of a trip with Sue and our boys and two other families. All seven of the kids on the trip were below the age of 6. Most had congregated around me

Twelve Tips that Save Kid Trips

1. Tell stories.
2. Team up with other families.
3. Ply them with treats.
4. Make yourself the mule.
5. Don't be a taskmaster.
6. Talk big, do small.
7. Buy the right gear.
8. Let them look the part.
9. Bring plenty of water.
10. Ban the sun.
11. Celebrate their achievements.
12. Be sure *you* have fun.

on one of our party's three rafts, where they sprawled beneath the hot sun, bored and irritable.

Up to that point, all of us had enjoyed the trip, kids and parents alike. We parents had minimized the time we and our kids had spent on the river each day by stretching what was normally a two-day trip into four days. During the potentially boring hours on the river, we'd held water fights, pulled the kids behind the rafts in inner tubes, conducted belly-flop contests off the sides of the rafts, and handed out cold drinks with liberal hands. But now, two hours from the takeout, the kids were tired of swimming, and the last of the cold drinks had long been drunk. We'd exited the sandstone canyon that marked most of our journey and instead were floating between broad, boring alfalfa fields. The characterless view and blazing sun had the kids growing crankier by the minute.

As I reclined among the kids at the front of the raft, they poked each other in the ribs and pinched each other's thighs to relieve their tedium. Soon fisticuffs would break out. It was up to me to come up with something, and fast.

I picked up an empty beer can from the floor of the raft and clicked its sides together experimentally. I spoke into the can's pop-top opening. "Testing one, two, three, four. Testing, testing." The kids stopped their squabbling and turned to me, attracted by the odd sound of my voice, nasal and metallic.

I had them. But what was I to do with them?

"Greetings," I addressed them, the can to my mouth like a microphone. "Welcome aboard the H.M.S. Razorback Sucker."

The microphone-can and my aluminumally enhanced voice gave me my identity: I was a tour guide.

With wide eyes and bouncing eyebrows, my free hand waving, I launched into a seat-of-the-pants tale about a pair of imagined brothers who once had lived in the ramshackle riverside mobile home, past which we happened to be floating at that very moment. The two brothers, Vinny and Victor, went on to have a slew of silly adventures around the world, the details of which I related in true tour-guide fashion over the course of the next 45 minutes.

When, finally, the takeout site hove into view, the kids turned away from me to hang over the front end of the raft and hungrily eye the cottonwood-shaded landing. I quickly brought Vinny and Victor home to a life of leisure in their weather-beaten trailer and ended my narration, crisis averted.

When situations such as the potential mutiny on the Colorado River confront you on the trips you take with your kids, you'll wish, as I did, you could just stick them in front of a DVD and relax. Such an opportunity, however, isn't possible in the outdoors. Instead, it'll be up to you to keep your kids occupied by whatever means you can come up with.

Trip Savers

Boredom, monotony, bad weather, tiredness, fear—any number of factors can take the glow off an outdoor adventure with kids. There's much you can do to keep things positive, however, including the following 12 tips that save kid trips.

TELL STORIES

Personal storytelling is fast becoming a lost art in our television-saturated society, but it's an art worth rediscovering if you want to have fun exploring the outdoors adventurously with your kids. Everybody loves a good story, kids most of all.

Storytelling is the primary weapon Sue and I use to fight boredom in the outdoors with our boys. While hiking along one trail or another, Taylor and Logan have heard most of the tales of Sue's and my pre-kid life together—how we met, the mountains we climbed, the trips we took, the jobs we worked. They've also heard capsulized versions of *Moby Dick*, *Tom Sawyer*, *Star Wars*,

> **Storytelling is an art worth rediscovering if you want to have fun exploring the outdoors adventurously with your kids.**

and *Jaws*—anything to keep their minds occupied and their feet moving.

TEAM UP WITH OTHER FAMILIES

Playmates and the resultant peer pressure they create are great for pushing your kids to keep moving through the boring, uncomfortable, or scary parts of outdoor adventures.

It's difficult to bring other kids along with you without their parents, however, because of the extra gear extra kids require. Better to find like-minded families and combine forces.

Many of the outdoor trips Sue and I take with our boys are with other families. The fun our boys have with other kids, and Sue and I with other parents, makes those trips truly enjoyable.

PLY THEM WITH TREATS

This is bribery, no more, no less. And it works.

The key to using this weapon effectively is to keep the treats hidden until you need them. Our boys know we generally have some sort of special treat along on the backcountry trips we take with them. Their anticipation of what that treat might be helps as much to keep them moving as the actual unveiling and partaking of the treat itself.

MAKE YOURSELF THE MULE

Successful outdoor adventures with children are all about keeping kids' levels of energy and enthusiasm up. That means not burdening them with gear.

As they grow older, your kids will want to carry a share of the load. When that time comes, let them. (Believe me, by then, you'll be more than happy to do so.) But don't overload them, and be prepared to take the load off their shoulders and put it back on yours when they begin to wear out.

Logan insisted on carrying his own tiny pack on the first family backpacking trip we took when he grew old enough to hike on his own. At the trailhead, Logan, then 4, proudly donned his 5-pound pack. He led the way up the trail until the pack became too much for him, at which point he turned it over to me. Unencumbered, he ran on up the trail while I strapped his pack atop my own. As I hoisted my pack back onto my shoulders, I glanced back down the trail. Through the trees, I could just make out the trail-head and parking area, about 100 yards away.

Don't be a Taskmaster

Sue and I have come to the conclusion that chores are for home. Trips into the back-country are demanding of youngsters in many ways. There's no need to add to those demands the added responsibility of doing chores.

Your goal is for your children to have fun on the outdoor adven-tures you under-take with them so they'll want to do more of the same with you in the future. One way to help guarantee your kids have fun is by declaring your outdoor adventures chore-free. Let your kids enjoy themselves on the outdoor adventures you take with them. If they want to help set up the tent or unload equipment from the car, fine. But if they'd rather play while you do the grunt work, so be it.

(Of course, things will change as your children mature. At a certain point, when they hit age 11 or 12 or so, requiring your kids' help on trips will be an important part of their maturation process, equally as important as not requiring it was when they were younger.)

TALK BIG, DO SMALL

As important as it is to pitch the incredulity of a trip to your kids in order to get them stoked to do it, it's just as important to choose adventures your kids can accomplish. It's far better to err on the side of conservatism than to end up tackling something your kids can't complete. If you take on a trip that's more than your kids can handle, they'll end up frustrated and less willing to head out with you again in the future.

Choose adventures your kids can accomplish.

If you recognize you've over-reached, don't be afraid to turn around or even call off an adventure right at the beginning. If the weather's bad or bugs are out or new boots are causing blisters, there'll always be another weekend.

USE THE RIGHT GEAR

Sue and I have no problem justifying the money we spend on the right equipment for the various outdoor sports we undertake with Taylor and Logan. We reason that if we took traditional vacations, we'd spend far more on Disneyland tickets, Universal Studios tours, and Sea World admissions than we'll ever spend on gear.

In many cases, it's only through the rental or purchase of specialized gear that you can even undertake various outdoor adventures with your kids.

For more information about gear, see Chapter 10, page 91.

LET THEM LOOK THE PART

Pride is a big part of success. If your kids are proud of how they look because you've dressed them well for the adventure at hand, they'll be less prone to quitting when the going gets tough.

Moreover, if you dress your kids in the right clothes for the outdoor sports you tackle with them, they'll be as comfortable and well-protected from the elements as the big-time athletes they'll look like.

BRING PLENTY OF WATER

Well-hydrated kids are content kids.

Sue often teases me about the extra liter of water I always throw in my pack (or Sue's, if I can get away with it) when we head out for a day with our boys. Still, every now and then, that liter proves handy, not in terms of saving a life, but by way of keeping our boys happily hydrated and thus excited for the next adventure when the time comes.

BAN THE SUN

Nothing saps the energy of children more than the sun beating down on their bare skin, yet I constantly see children in the backcountry on sunny days wearing sleeveless shirts and no hats.

Shielding your kids from the sun makes sense simply in terms of minimizing the risk that they'll contract skin cancer when they get older. Moreover, by keeping the sun off your kids, you'll conserve their energy. Energetic kids are happy kids, and happy kids make for successful outdoor adventures.

CELEBRATE THEIR ACHIEVEMENTS

The best thing about kids and outdoor action sports is that there are no winners and losers. The whole point of outdoor sports is simply to have fun.

Still, when Taylor or Logan are successful at something in the outdoors, Sue and I make a point of recognizing it, most often in the form of a celebratory meal out as a family.

When your kids reach their goals in the outdoors—when they top out on a climbing route or summit a peak, when they hike 5 miles or 3 or 1, when they run their first Class II or III rapid—champion their success. More than anything else you can do, celebrating your kids' outdoor achievements will keep them coming back for more.

BE SURE *YOU* HAVE FUN

No matter what goes wrong during the outdoor adventures you tackle with your kids, keep your focus on the journey, on having fun.

Kids take their cues from their parents, especially when they're trying something that's new and strange to them. Come what may, if you have fun outdoor adventuring with your kids, they'll have fun with you.

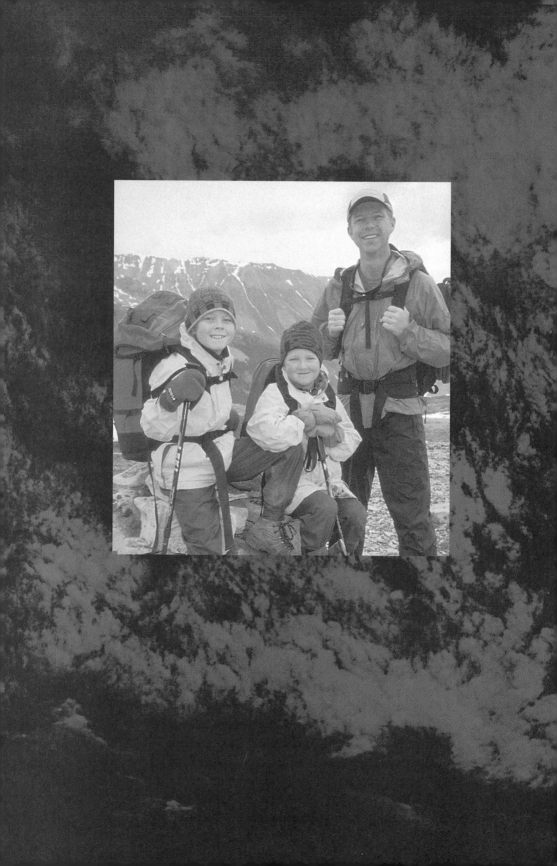

9 Keeping Your Kids Safe

Teamed with our friends Mark and Jeanne Pastore and their two kids one early-spring weekend, Sue and I and our boys, then 9 and 7, headed up Cottonwood Reef into a gathering storm. We knew we might well get wet during our off-trail overnighter on the reef, a canted ridge of sandstone in far western Colorado. If we'd known what we really were in for that night, however, I doubt we would ever have left our cars.

Cottonwood Reef slants upward and to the west at a 20-degree angle. From its highest point, it plummets 600 feet straight down to Cottonwood Wash below. We planned to pitch our tents on the slickrock lip of the reef overlooking the cliffs, canyons, and piñon-covered mesas beyond.

The wind picked up as we climbed the tilted slickrock. As we neared the top of the ridge, the wind, coming up and over the escarpment's flat western face, was blowing even harder. There was no way we could pitch our tents anywhere near the windswept precipice.

The clouds thickened and the wind grew to a howl as we retreated back down the slanted rock, searching for a site to erect our tents. Trouble was, everything below the lip of the reef was set at an angle. At one point, we left our packs on the tilted rock and set off in different directions, searching for potential tent sites. When we returned, our packs were gone. The gale-force gusts had sent them tumbling far down the slope and into a narrow slot in the sloping slickrock, where we eventually found them.

The only flat, wind-protected site in the area was at the bottom of the minor drainage that gathered runoff water from the surrounding portion of the reef and channeled it down the sloping sandstone. We had a choice: We could pitch our tents in the drainage, or we could give up and return to our cars.

We debated. The clouds were gathering, but it wasn't raining. Besides, even during the worst spring storms, little precipitation tended to fall here in the high desert.

We put up our tents in the drainage, cooked dinner, and settled in for the night.

I awoke in full darkness to the soft patter of a few raindrops on the tent. I checked my watch.

"What time is it?" Sue asked, already awake beside me.

"A little after 3."

"What do you think?"

"What do *you* think?" I responded nervously, imagining raindrops gathering and pooling and heading down the drainage toward us.

Over the next few minutes, as the kids slept on, Sue and I talked things over with Mark and Jeanne through the walls of our side-by-side tents. The rain remained light. Then, like turning off a faucet, it quit.

The four of us expressed our mutual relief and went back to sleep.

Twenty minutes later, the rain started up again as quickly as it had ended. This time it came hard and fast. Large drops pounded our tents. By the time Jeanne, Mark, Sue, and I pulled on our rain gear and headlamps and scrambled out into the deluge, water already was trickling down the drainage and around our tents. We rousted the kids, dressed them in their rain gear, and tucked them beneath an overhang while we stowed our sleeping bags, pads, and tents.

The eight of us put our backs to the wind and set off down the sandstone ridge beneath the steady downpour. It was 4 in the morning, and it was bone-chillingly cold. Jeanne, Mark, Sue, and I were miserable. The kids, however, fairly skipped down the slickrock, the beams of their headlamps dancing in the rain. They'd never gotten to bail out of a camp in the middle of the night before, and they were ecstatic about getting to do so.

The kids' excitement quickly infected us parents, and the eight of us completed the hike off the ridge in fine form. We arrived back at our cars beneath dawning skies and headed to the nearest restaurant for breakfast, then home for a long midday nap.

Middle Ground

There are two ways to look at our aborted Cottonwood Reef trip.

On one hand, some could reasonably argue, we should never have pitched our tents in the drainage that evening.

On the other hand, others could argue, we were fine pitching our tents where we did, and we shouldn't have broken camp so hastily. (As it turned out, the rain began to let up shortly after we started down the ridge. It had stopped by the time we reached our cars. No doubt the trickle of water in the drainage remained just that.)

Between those two extremes, I prefer to defend our middle-ground approach. Yes, we pitched our tents in a drainage. But we did so knowing the drainage ended only 200 yards above us at the top of the ridge—not enough distance to result in much runoff. Moreover, we broke camp as soon as the rain became heavy.

When it comes to safety, participating in outdoor sports with kids has much to do with finding middle ground—that is, with practicing common sense.

Jack Turner, producer of the televised *Next Snow Search* competition for kids, and his wife took their children through Class V rapids and past numerous keeper holes on a private-party rafting trip down the Grand Canyon when their kids were 6 and 8.

"Some people would say we took unnecessary chances with them," Turner says. "But we were careful. And what we did with them was real."

Turner doesn't deny that the pastimes he and his wife pursue with their kids involve danger. "Sure, there's a chance our kids could get hurt," he says. "It just depends on how you want to live your life. My wife and I aren't risk-averse people. In my opinion, risk is what makes people really live."

Turner says his kids live an "adventure lifestyle." "We go on raft trips, ski trips, you name it," he says. "Last summer we did a 40-mile, six-day, llama-supported trip into the middle of nowhere."

The result? Because Turner and his wife are willing to expose their children to a modicum of risk in the outdoors, says Turner, his kids "may not really know it, but they exude a sense of adventure, a sense of confidence."

> Often, the most dangerous aspect of an outdoor adventure is the drive to the put-in, cliff face, beach, or trailhead.

Not that Dangerous

There are those who argue that the potential dangers of outdoor sports make them too risky to take on with children. You're backpacking into the wilderness far from medical care with your kids, running rapids, climbing cliffs, jumping logs on bikes, encountering riptides, and dealing with lightning, avalanches, rattlesnakes.

Yet for all the concern some people have about parents like me and Turner taking our kids into the outdoors, or about the X Game-like TV shows and all the radical pictures in the out-there magazines, outdoor sports aren't all that dangerous. In reality, the most dangerous aspect of an outdoor adventure is often the drive to the put-in, cliff face, beach, or trailhead.

On one of the days I spoke with Kristine Jackson, she was running the car shuttle while Eric, Emily, and Dane ran a remote and challenging stretch of whitewater.

"Right now, my children are having an incredible wilderness experience," Kristine told me. "They're with their father and they're doing something that they'll be really proud of—and something that's far safer than if they were to drive to the video-game center at the mall."

Even so, Kristine says, people often tell her she's crazy for allowing her children to run big water with their father.

"I'd be considered borderline irresponsible if one of my kids got hurt kayaking," she says. "Yet people don't think twice about throwing their kids in the car for no apparent reason, to go shopping or whatever. And if they get in a wreck and their kids get hurt, nobody would dream of saying to them, 'Did you really need to go to the mall?'"

Kristine says she believes kids who participate in so-called "extreme" sports actually end up living safer lives than those who don't. "Any kids in any extreme sports are already doing something that most people consider dangerous," she says. "That ends up keeping them away from things that really are dangerous, like drugs and alcohol. They don't need to experiment with those sorts of things because they know what real risk is all about."

Balance

Keeping your kids safe in the outdoors is all about finding balance, about being conservatively adventurous with them, about opting to bail from a campsite when odds are you don't really need to. It's about being careful, and remembering that the whole point of what you're doing is to have fun with your kids—and there's no fun in putting your kids' lives at risk.

As Kristine Jackson puts it: "Eric understands how precious each day of kayaking with our children is.

85

Although from the outside looking in it may be hard to see, he's actually very careful with Emily and Dane."

The best way to determine your comfort level when it comes to adventure and perceived danger is to choose the sports you try with your kids carefully and with open eyes.

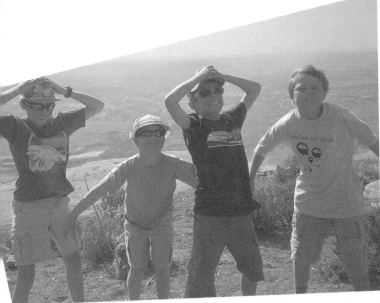

In the early 1980s, I gazed at the pictures in the pages of *Climbing* and *Rock and Ice* magazines of rock jocks climbing incredible cliff faces, and I decided I wanted to be one of them. I signed up for a climbing course, learned the basics, and teamed up with more experienced partners for climbs near Albuquerque, New Mexico, where Sue and I then lived. I joined the Albuquerque Mountain Rescue Team and attended training exercises where I practiced knot tying, Z-pulley systems, and stretcher-belay scenarios.

The more I climbed, the more I found that the complexities of placing protection and setting anchors overwhelmed me. It dawned on me that all my fellow climbers were seriously intelligent people who made their livings as scientists, engineers, and computer programmers. And then there was me—the generally dazed, always confused writer.

Given enough time, I came to realize, I would eventually kill myself if I kept climbing, and I'd likely take whoever was at the other end of the rope with me. I simply didn't— and still don't—have the focused, detail-oriented brain rock climbing demands of its participants.

I never did grace the pages of any climbing magazines. I am, however, alive today, and there's something to be said for that. I gave up climbing because I recognized my limits. It turns out I'm fine at slogging. I'm a good hiker, a fine backpacker, a solid mountaineer. I handle altitude well. I enjoy the challenges presented by glacier travel and high, walk-up peaks.

Just don't let me lead anything vertical. My brain, I realized (fortunately in time) isn't made for the kind of thinking demanded of lead climbers on traditional big-wall routes. Even so, that realization hasn't kept me from introducing Taylor and Logan to rock climbing. Top-rope climbing—climbing short rock faces while safely attached to ropes solidly anchored from above—is simply too enjoyable to keep from them.

Providing your children a repertoire of outdoor sports is only fair to them.

Today, Taylor, at age 11, loves the sport, while Logan, at age 8, isn't yet as taken with climbing. Still, the basics of climbing (and the fun of it—grabbing for holds, dangling from a rope, swinging out from a wall high above the ground) are part of Logan's outdoor repertoire.

Providing your children a repertoire is only fair to them. Don't limit your children to just one outdoor sport because it happens to be the one you do and therefore it's the one you think you'll be able to keep your kids safe at. As long as you're careful and on top of things, you'll be able to try all sorts of outdoor sports safely with your kids. In return, they'll be able to choose from among those sports and pursue further the ones that interest them most, rather than being condemned to do only "your" sport until they grow up and head out on their own.

Dive in Safely

Over the course of his 30-year career, Jon Ross of High Angle Adventures has taught more than 15,000 adults and children to climb at eastern New York's Shawangunk Cliffs. Ross says he's learned over the years that preadolescent kids are far more conservative than most adults realize.

When Something Goes Wrong

My wife, Sue, is an emergency physician. As such, you'd think she'd be pretty uptight about the first-aid kit she brings on backcountry excursions. If you thought that, however, you'd be wrong.

Based on her years of treating patients injured in backcountry accidents at our local emergency room, Sue's message regarding backcountry first aid is straightforward: If an injury can be handled easily in the backcountry, by all means handle it.

■ Clean a minor cut, squeeze on some antibiotic ointment, and stick a Band-Aid over it.

■ Use ibuprofen or acetaminophen for minor aches and pains.

■ Cover blisters with moleskin.

■ Carry an epinephrine pen if you or your children have a history of allergic reactions to bee stings or specific foods, or if you don't know yet regarding your children.

■ Use diphenhydramine (Benadryl) to minimize insect-bite and poison-ivy reactions.

But if an injury calls for more major attention, Sue echoes most, if not all, emergency physicians when she recommends a single course of action: Get the patient to professional medical care as quickly as possible.

The most likely major injury you or one of your children will incur in the backcountry is a bad cut. Some medical professionals, particularly those who make their livings teaching wilderness survival courses, teach the cleaning and stitching up or packing with gauze of such lacerations in the field.

The reality, however, is that adequately cleaning a serious wound is impossible in the field, where a sterile environment doesn't exist. Packing or stitching closed an inadequately cleaned wound may well lead to serious infection. Better to apply pressure to the open wound and get the patient to a medical facility.

The answer, then, isn't to put together a huge first-aid kit with grand plans to use it for emergencies in the field. The answer, rather, is to always have a plan as to how best to get an injured patient out of the field as quickly and efficiently as possible in the event of such an emergency. That's the best first aid you can bring with you on any journey into the backcountry with your children.

"But that doesn't mean they have good judgment," he's quick to point out. "Judgment is the result of repeated experience."

Ross says preadolescence is a great time for kids to get that repeated experience and grounding in good judgment—before their teenage years and the sense of immortality that inevitably accompanies that period of life.

Hence, when it comes to outdoor adventuring with kids, the key is to dive in—but to do so in a way that is as safe as possible for you and your kids alike. For some sports, that may mean searching out and paying for guides and good, solid instruction. For others, it may mean finding parents already doing the sport that interests you with their kids and tagging along with them. For still others, it may just mean taking your time and edging your way in, all on your own. Ultimately, though, there's no reason not to try a variety of outdoor sports with your kids. That's how they'll grow to be well-rounded adults who love and respect the outdoors.

Is there a risk that your kids will get hurt in the process? Sure. Is that small risk worth it? No question.

"I can guarantee you that kids will get hurt and some might even die from action sports in the future," says Turner, the producer of television's *Next Snow Search* competition. "But a million more kids who don't participate in action sports will eventually die from their sedentary lifestyle, from laying around on the couch and getting overweight, from diabetes and heart attacks and whatever else."

Safety concerns fully acknowledged, Turner echoes all the parents I know who participate in outdoor sports with their kids. "You can either live under a rock and hide from life, or you can go out there with your kids and do it," he says.

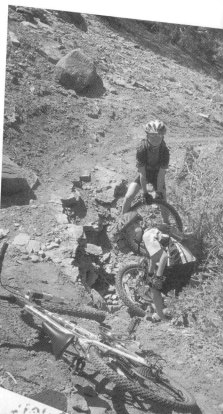

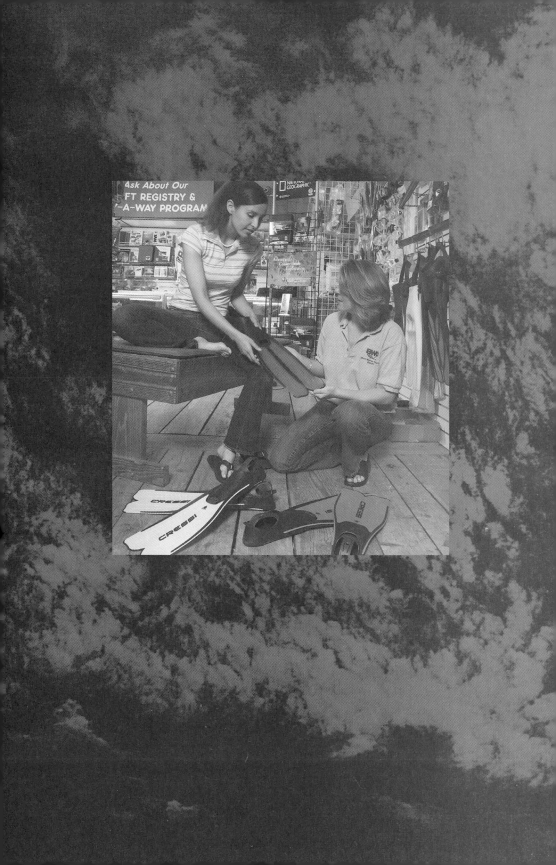

10 Gear: The Right Stuff for Your Kids

Every parent knows that children are gear intensive from the minute they're born. Things only get worse when you introduce your kids to the world of outdoor action sports. How to deal with all the gear you'll need for the sports you try with your kids? Piece by piece, sport by sport, and, unfortunately, dollar by dollar.

The chapters on particular sports in the remainder of this book include gear discussions for each of those sports. This chapter deals with cost, size, and type of kid outdoor gear in general, as well as how, when, and where to buy affordable, quality gear for your children.

Cost

You may be concerned that the gear you'll need in order to expose your children to just one outdoor sport—much less several—will cost you a fortune. And while it's true that buying outdoor gear for your kids can be expensive, it doesn't have to be.

There are two ways to affordably check out a new outdoor sport with your kids: rent, or buy cheap or used gear. Rental, lesser-quality, and used gear is readily available for most outdoor sports. It makes good financial sense to begin there and buy new, high-quality gear only for sports you and your kids want to pursue further.

Take bodyboarding, for example. If you're planning a vacation to a beach with good waves, you can count on

91

finding rental bodyboards when you arrive. Conversely, for about the same price as renting a good-quality board for a day, you can buy a cheap bodyboard that'll last a vacation or, if you're lucky, two.

And if you enjoy your vacation so much you decide to hit a wave-play beach every year? *That's* the time to invest in good boards, as well as fins and rash-guard shirts.

Size

Correctly sized gear is critical to kids having fun in the outdoors. Fortunately, many outdoor-gear manufacturers are recognizing that there's money to be made off the many youngsters now being turned on to outdoor sports by their parents, and they're responding accordingly. These days, many outdoor-equipment manufacturers produce high-quality, kid-size gear:

- For more than a decade, climbing-gear companies such as Trango and Black Diamond have made harnesses for tiny climbers. Logan first climbed in his Trango harness at age 3.

- Innovations and improvements in suspension, gearing, and braking constantly trickle down to kid-size mountain bikes.

- Telemark boot maker Garmont now produces a plastic telemark boot model for kids. Named the Teledactyl, the boot, predictably, is available only in kid-appealing blaze orange.

- Kids' helmets, hiking boots, sun hats, sun shirts, UV-blocking sunglasses, and waterproof/breathable jackets and pants—all are widely available today.

Trouble is, while gear for kids is almost as expensive as adult gear, kids don't get a heck of a lot of use out of their gear before they outgrow it. In response, you may be tempted to buy gear for your kids that's too big so they'll use it longer and you'll "get your money's worth" out of it. Don't allow yourself to fall into that trap. Instead, when it comes time to switch from rental or low-end to high-end kid gear for a particular sport, buy the right size. Your kids will be the direct beneficiaries of your largesse.

Rather than trying to stretch your dollars by buying gear that's too big, try shopping the used market and end-of-season sales. In so doing, you'll be able to buy high-end gear at good prices and sell it for not much less when your kids have outgrown it. Admittedly, such a process requires more work than simply buying what you want for your kids the moment you and they want it. But other than the initial investment—much of which you'll eventually recoup—buying high-end gear on the cheap enables you to outfit your kids for any number of sports almost for free.

If you buy high-end gear on the cheap and resell it when your kids have outgrown the gear, you'll recoup much of your initial investment.

Lightweight Gear

Many of the sports discussed in this book involve camping—near a car during a rock climbing trip, near a river during a rafting trip, or near a lake during a paddle-and-portage canoeing trip—so it's worth a quick look here at overnight gear as it relates to various outdoor sports.

The marketing mantra in the outdoor industry for the last few years has been to switch to the latest in lightweight gear. At first, I saw that marketing scheme as similar to fashion designers raising and lowering skirt lengths—an opportunity to get everyone to buy a new round of gear. Turns out I was wrong.

My first lightweight gear purchase was a down sleeping bag that uses a super-thin nylon sheath, stuffs down to the size of a liter bottle, and weighs only 2 pounds. The bag more than halved the weight and space requirements of the old down bag I'd sworn by for 20 years. I followed up that purchase by buying an ultralight, 2-pound backpack to replace my old 7-pound pack.

In two purchases, I dropped my backpacking weight requirements by 7 pounds. I was hooked.

Since then, I've gradually added a lightweight tent, the super-light MSR Miox water purifier (www.msrcorp.com), and a feather-light propane stove to my backpacking gear.

The ultralight mantra applies to more than just backpacking. It's worth applying to the gear your kids use for the various outdoor action sports they tackle with you. The lighter their gear, the freer they are to move and perform whatever outdoor sport they're attempting. That means they'll be more apt to enjoy the sport and pursue it in the future.

The mantra also is worth applying to your car-camping gear purchases. Buying light means you'll minimize the amount of weight you'll have to haul from the garage to your car and from your car to your campsite each time you go camping.

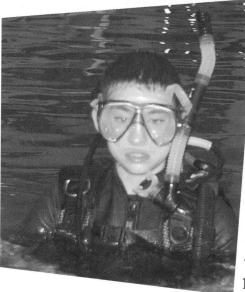

The amount Sue and I have spent on lightweight camping gear, about $1000, is less than the cost of a single trip to Disneyland, and already has made possible years of enjoyable backcountry trips with our boys.

For more information on light-weight camping gear, check out www.backpacker.com, www.back-packing.net, and www.backpack-inglight.com. Though aimed at the backpacking crowd, all three sites offer reviews of light-weight gear that works as well for car and boat camping as it does for backpacking.

What to Buy

Start with the internet when you attempt to figure out what to buy for any new sport you want to try with your kids. I'm consistently surprised by how much I can learn about a particular sport and the gear it requires simply by typing the name of the sport into an internet search engine and surfing the results.

Once you've done your initial research online, buy locally if you're buying new and your budget will allow it. Although the web is great for getting started, you'll learn much more from salespeople who know the gear they sell. When it comes to outdoor sports that are new to you, that knowledge is worth the premium brick-and-mortar stores must charge for their gear in season.

Moreover, if you're ahead of the game, the fact that brick-and-mortar stores must unload their stock to make room for the next season's stuff makes for killer end-of-season deals.

As for buying used outdoor gear over the internet, caveat emptor. When it comes to outdoor gear, the term

Where to Find It

After you do some preliminary learning on the internet, outdoor sporting goods stores that carry gear for the sport you're planning to try with your children are the logical place to start looking for the kid gear you'll need. Other places to look, especially if you're trying to save money, include:

- Gear swaps (held annually by many outdoor gear retailers)
- Second-hand sporting goods stores
- Thrift stores in outdoor-oriented towns
- Garage sales
- Outfitters replacing their kid gear
- Online outdoor gear outlet stores, including www.rei-outlet.com, www.sierratradingpost.com, and the closeout section of www.campmor.com
- Online price search engines such as www.froogle.com

Note, too, that brick-and-mortar outdoor gear retailers (and online ones as well) must hold sales to clear out their inventories at the end of each season to make way for the next season's wares. If you're willing to take a chance on how big you think your children will be in a few months, you can save big bucks by shopping such end-of-season sales.

"used" has a wide range of meanings. I buy used outdoor gear sight unseen for Taylor and Logan only rarely and only when the price is more than right and I'm sure the gear I'm buying is in like-new condition. One of the best ways I've found for buying used gear online is from outfitters and rental shops updating their fleets of children's equipment. Such gear generally is of high quality and in the shape claimed by the outfitters, who face the prospect of losing future business if they misrepresent the condition of their wares.

HELMETS

Most outdoor sport injuries are of the minor, scrapes-and-bruises variety. Of the major injuries that result from outdoor sports, broken bones heal, but broken heads may not. That's why no piece of equipment is more important to you as a parent introducing your kids to outdoor sports than helmets. Nor is any piece of equipment more seemingly overpriced—until you come around to thinking of helmets not as pieces of equipment, but as individual insurance policies made of brightly colored plastic. As insurance policies, helmets are remarkably cheap and entirely worthwhile.

Sue and I enjoy trying to save money when it comes to buying outdoor gear for our boys—except when it comes to helmets. For everything other than helmets, we haunt second-hand sporting goods stores, gear swaps, thrift stores, and garage sales. But we're willing to pay whatever's necessary to protect our boys' noggins. In fact, the high-tech composite kayaking helmet we recently bought for Logan at our local kayaking store cost more than his boat, which we found at a gear swap.

Though multisport helmets exist, you're better off buying the right helmet for each sport. It's all about putting your money in the right place: protecting your kids' heads. Kid-size kayaking helmets are designed to function when wet, snow-sport helmets to keep kids' ears warm, and bike helmets to keep kids' heads cool; each type is specific to its sport and should be purchased that way.

CLOTHING

High-quality clothing is as helpful to kids in the outdoors as it is to adults. Though Sue and I work at saving money on all the outdoor clothing we buy for Taylor and Logan, we don't flinch at paying full price every now and then for whatever clothes our boys require to look the part and comfortably tackle whatever adventure we've cooked up for them next.

> **As insurance policies, helmets are remarkably cheap and entirely worthwhile.**

You'll find deals on general outdoor clothing for kids in the catalogs and on the websites of Sierra Trading Post (www.sierratradingpost.com) and Campmor (www.campmor.com).

WATER STORAGE

Sooner rather than later, you'll begin having trouble carrying all the water you and your kids will drink during a round of adventuring in the outdoors. The answer is to outfit your kids with Camelbak or equivalent water packs. Kids love wearing water packs. You'll love that they love wearing them because these hydration systems get the water weight off your back and onto theirs. Camelbak (www.camelbak.com) makes several kid-size water packs for children as young as 5.

SLEEPING BAGS AND COATS

Though synthetic insulation continues to get better, it still doesn't beat down's weight-to-warmth ratio. In addition, down remains far more stuffable than synthetics. The two big advantages of synthetic fill over down are that it retains its insulating abilities when wet, and it dries far more quickly than down.

If you anticipate doing most of your camping with your kids in wet or damp conditions, synthetic-filled sleeping bags and coats may be the way to go. In drier climates, down wins. Moreover, if, like me and many other parents, you head outdoors with your kids only when relatively dry weather is forecast, down will work for you even in parts of the country that often are rainy.

Many manufacturers make super-light down sleeping bags for adults, but children's bags come only in synthetic. Synthetic-filled kids' bags cost less than $100 and weigh little more than 2 pounds, but they don't compress easily. For that added benefit, you'll be faced with investing in an ultralight short adult bag filled with down, though such a bag will run you $200 or more and won't stand up to much abuse.

Kelty (www.kelty.com) and many other companies make affordable synthetic-filled sleeping bags for children. Marmot (www.marmot.com), Western Mountaineering (www.westernmountaineering.com), and several other companies make ultralight down bags in adult sizes.

Sweater-weight, synthetic-filled coats work well for children. However, the reduced bulk of down makes it the top choice for children's big winter coats. The stuffability of down also makes it a good choice for kids' vests, brought along on outdoor trips as an extra insulation layer.

Most high-end outdoor clothing manufacturers have children's lines, including The North Face (www.thenorth-face.com), Patagonia (www.patagonia.com), and REI (www.rei.com). In addition, Campmor (www.campmor.com) carries a perfectly service-able line of affordable outdoor cloth-ing for children that bears its company label.

RAINWEAR

Gore-Tex remains the best waterproof/breathable rain-wear fabric on the market. However, new waterproof/breathable fabrics that lean closer to the waterproof end of the spectrum than the breathable end are cutting into Gore-Tex's market share. Those fabrics have the advantage of being far less expensive than Gore-Tex.

For more information and to look at specific rain jackets and rain pants for kids, see the outdoor clothing websites for REI, Patagonia, and The North Face. For inexpensive children's rainwear, check out Red Ledge (www.redledge.com) as well as Campmor.

SLEEPING PADS

Nothing beats Therm-a-Rest sleeping pads (www.ther-marest.com) for comfort, weight, and compressibility. Sue and I carry four super-light, three-quarter-length pads when we're camping with Taylor and Logan. We carry L-shaped foam Crazy Creek chairs (www.crazycreek.com) for simple, on-the-ground seating and, when sleeping, as padding for our feet where our three-quarter-length pads end.

TENTS

Tent choices break down between traveling with one large family tent, or using two or more two-man tents.

Some families, ours included, enjoy sleeping together in one tent. The best, though far from perfect, lightweight family tent I've found is the Nuk Tuk, made by Dana Design (www.danadesign.com). The Nuk Tuk is an update of Black Diamond's venerable pyramid-shaped Megamid tarp-tent (www.bdel.com), which Sue and I favored before Taylor and Logan came along. (Super-light tarp-tents like the Megamid are popular with the go-light crowd. Such shelters work well for adults, but the migratory patterns of sleeping children are best kept in check by the confines of traditional tents with attached walls and floors.)

The Nuk Tuk weighs only 6 pounds, yet its floor measures 8 feet by 8 feet, room enough to sleep four comfortably. The tent is so tall at its center pole that youngsters can stand inside it while getting dressed.

Without its fly, the Nuk Tuk boasts an all-mosquito-netting inner tent for stargazing and staying cool on warm clear nights.

The disadvantages of the Nuk Tuk are directly related to its advantages. Because its large size is supported by a single center pole, the tent's fly tends to droop when wet. Also, finding a level spot 8 feet by 8 feet in the backcountry sometimes can be difficult. Finally, because of its large size and all-netting interior, the Nuk Tuk is not a warm tent, and because of its height, it catches a lot of wind.

Some people dislike tents such as the Nuk Tuk because they aren't freestanding. I've never been bothered by that

> Tent choices break down between traveling with one large family tent, or using two or more two-man tents.

fact. When faced with a tent site not friendly to tent stakes, it's easy to slide sticks through the corner loops of a non-freestanding tent, pile rocks on the sticks, and—voilà—a tent that stands on its own.

Rather than sleep in one large tent, many families camp with two or more two-person tents. Sue and I favor the use of two small tents over the Nuk Tuk for family trips into the high country where cold and wind are significant factors. We use the pair of two-man tents we carry on such trips only for sleeping. In addition to the two tents, we carry a Megamid for cooking and congregating out of the weather during morning and evening hours.

There are a number of high-quality, affordable two-man tents on the market in the sub 4-pound range. One, the Firstlight by Black Diamond, weighs 2.5 pounds. Sue and I and our boys use and like the 3-pound cousin of the Firstlight, the Lighthouse, with its easy-entry side-wall door. See REI's website (www.rei.com) for a detailed tent overview.

Today's super-light LED headlamps are the perfect camp toys for kids.

STOVES

The first mini cook stove I ever owned, back in my Boy Scout days, was a pocket-size aluminum job fueled by a small butane canister. In the decades that followed, I joined the masses and moved on to various versions of white-gas and multi-fuel stoves—until, lo and behold, pocket-size canister stoves came roaring back into fashion.

Though they have their drawbacks, today's canister stoves are widely regarded as the best option for use in spring, summer, and fall—the seasons you'll be camping with your kids—because they're lightweight and easy to use.

There are dozens of canister stoves on the market, but the smallest is the 3-ounce Brunton Optimus Crux (www.brunton.com), which folds in half and tucks away in the concave base of its fuel tank.

LIGHTS

Today's super-light LED headlamps are the perfect camp toys for kids. The amount of light they emit is adequate for night hiking and evening play near camp. The LED lights shine brightly for up to 30 hours on a single set of AAA batteries.

Petzl's (www.petzl.com) 3-ounce Tikka and its cousins have been the leaders in this field for several years, though a number of other companies make high-quality LED headlamps as well.

PACKS

As with kid-size sleeping bags, the ultralight craze hasn't yet extended to kid-size backpacks. As a result, children's backpacks available today weigh 3.5 to a whopping 6 pounds—as opposed to only 2 pounds for a variety of ultra-light adult packs now on the market.

Rather than saddle Taylor and Logan with heavy kid packs, Sue and I have purchased for them the small women's version of the popular ultralight Ghost backpack made by Mountainsmith (www.mountain-smith.com). The women's short-torso version of the Ghost is known as the Seraph. It costs only a little more than kid-specific packs, weighs just 2 pounds, and boasts a generous 2000-cubic-inch capacity.

The Seraph is just small enough to fit Logan at age 8. It fits 11-year-old Taylor well. Both boys use their Seraphs for multiday backpacking trips and as gear, food, and clothing haulers for rock climbing and fly-fishing day trips.

Like Taylor and Logan, Sue and I use and enjoy the panel-loading Ghost packs for backpacking. Our full-size Ghosts are so light and comfortable that we use them rather than daypacks for dayhiking and peak bagging as well. Mountainsmith's line of ultralight packs was one of the earliest on the market; a number of companies now produce high-quality ultralight packs.

Because they're shaved of needless add-ons in order to save weight, ultralight packs cost much less than heavier, full-featured packs.

FOOTWEAR

Though manufacturers make all-leather hiking boots for children, Sue and I and other parents we know buy leather-and-fabric children's boots because they're less expensive than all-leather models.

Unlike all-leather boots, leather-and-fabric boots are not waterproof. I've found, however, that if Taylor and Logan are going to get their feet wet, they're usually going to get them *very* wet—by slipping off a rock into a creek, falling off a log into a lake, or simply hiking through a downpour. In those cases, their feet are going to get soaked no matter what type of boot they're wearing.

If you plan to hike extensively in the wet Cascades or the Northeast, all-leather or Gore-Tex-sock kid boots may be worth their added expense because dry-toed children are happy children. For hiking in drier climates, leather-and-fabric boots should be adequate.

The most widely available and affordable children's boot brand is Hi-Tec (www.hi-tec.com), carried by virtually every shoe retailer on the planet. Use of a price-based internet search engine will reveal sale prices on Hi-Tec children's boots at a variety of online retailers.

Keen (www.keenfootwear.com), Teva (www.teva.com), and a number of other manufacturers make sandal-style water-sport footwear in kid sizes.

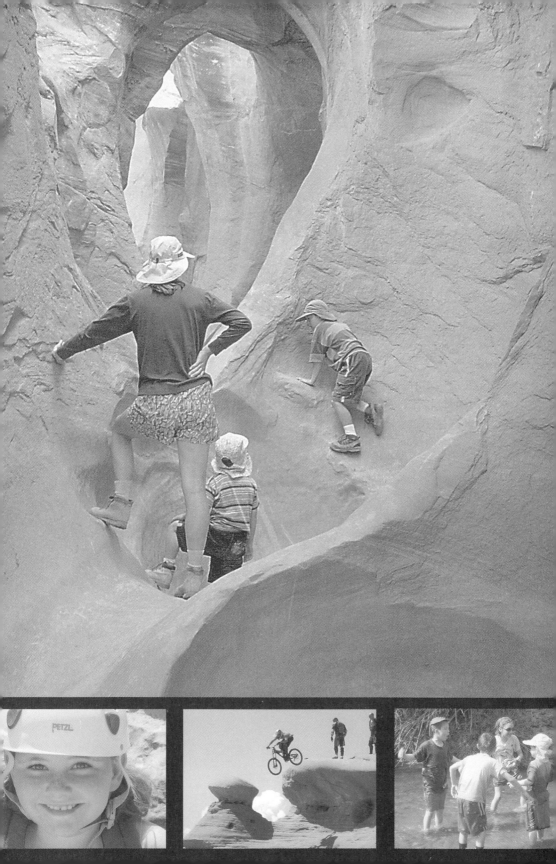

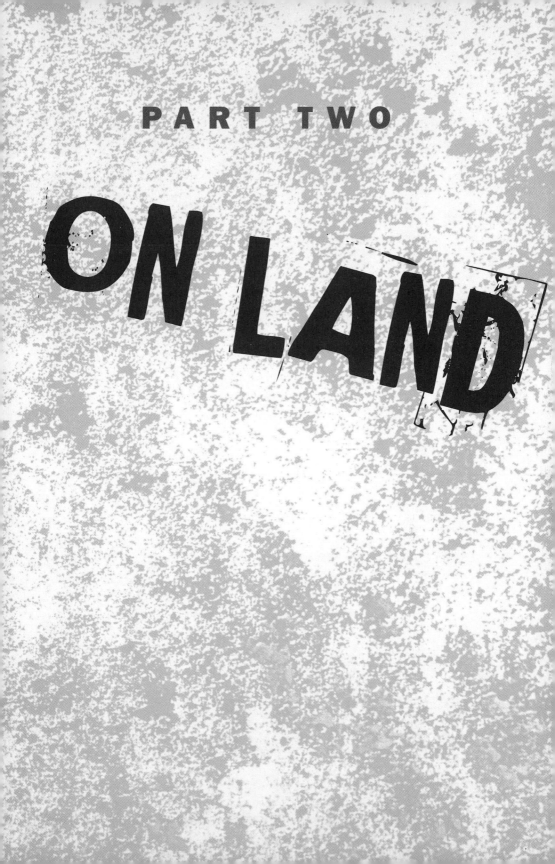

PART TWO

ON LAND

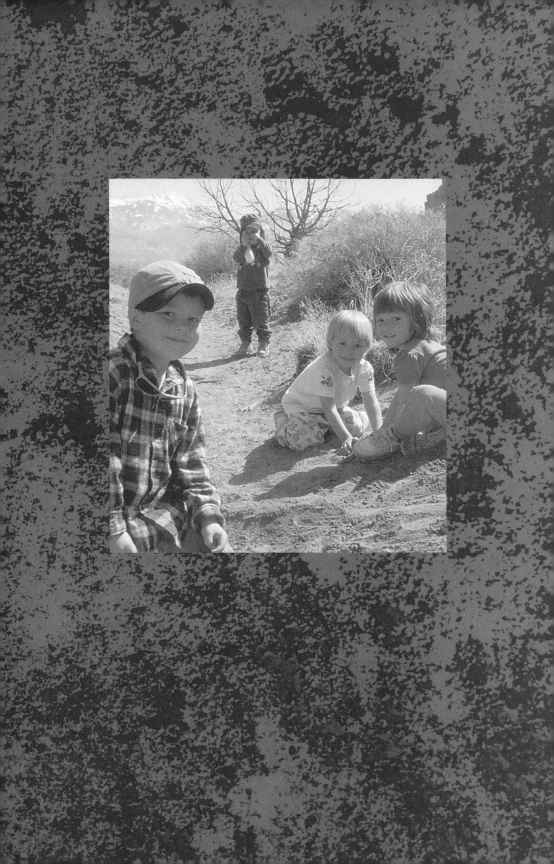

11 Extreme and Not-so-Extreme Dayhiking

D ayhiking is the easiest activity you can tackle in the outdoors with your kids. You can hold their hands and explore the banks of a creek when they're toddlers, play chase with them in the forest when they're 2, and complete hikes of a mile or two with them when they're 3.

Until age 4 or so, children love the simple act of walking in the woods—an act that gets them comfortable in the outdoors and ready to tackle more active forms of outdoor play in years to come. Beyond age 4, however, most kids need some encouragement when it comes to dayhiking. One of the best forms of encouragement is simply to up the dayhiking ante with your kids by tackling other forms of hiking with them, including geocaching, orienteering, trail running, and snowshoeing.

The Dreaded Dayhike

When Taylor and Logan were little, they had no choice but to come with me when I ran errands around town as part of my at-home-dad duties. The boys quickly came to despise this chore nearly as much as I did (and still do). They refused to get in the car when I so much as mentioned what came to be known in our family as the "E" word.

As a defense mechanism, I came up with a new expression each time I faced running errands with the boys.

107

Rather than "run errands," Taylor, Logan, and I "explored town." We went out to "forage" at the grocery store. We participated in "races," "endurance rallies," and "timed events" to see how many stores we could hit in an hour. We became "spies" casing the dentist's office and "barbarians" planning an assault on the hardware store.

The result? I still disliked running errands, but I got them done. And the boys enjoyed participating in these new adventures.

When the boys were old enough to begin hiking, they quickly learned to dislike the term "dayhiking" as much as they hated the term "errands." What Sue and I saw as a relaxing day in the woods, the boys saw as drudgery. And who could blame them? From the boys' perspective, dayhiking was a fancy word for forced march. They would much rather stay home and play in the yard than put one foot in front of the other over and over and over again. When Sue and I managed to drag the boys to a trailhead, they wanted to stay right there beside the car, playing basketball using wads of paper and the trailhead trash can as a basket.

Sue and I banished the term "dayhike" from our parenting lexicon as quickly as we had the term "errand." We no longer spoke with the boys of going out for a dayhike. Rather, we took them to "explore" a place they'd never visited. We went to "skip rocks" at a lake that just happened to be a mile's hike from where we parked. We went "bouldering" on rock faces that, likewise, were reached via hiking trails. We went on "reconnaissance missions" and "search-and-rescue efforts"—anything but dreaded dayhikes.

The Basics

- There's no easier way to begin exploring the outdoors with your kids than dayhiking.

- When your kids clamor for more than just dayhiking—but you'd like to keep doing it with them—you can up the ante by taking them dayhiking in the form of geocaching, orienteering, nature-game playing, and trail running.

- "Extreme" dayhiking in the form of off-trail and off-season hikes and explorations is another way to expand your opportunities to dayhike with your children as they grow older.

Our ploy worked. The boys had fun on our various excursions, and Sue and I had fun dayhiking with them.

First Hikes

In addition to coming up with camouflage descriptions for what really is dayhiking, you can tackle several activities in the outdoors with your kids that approximate dayhiking and that your kids will love. As detailed later in this chapter, those activities include geocaching, orienteering, trail running, and snowshoeing. You also can add spice to dayhikes with your kids by participating with them in nature-appreciation activities and games during your hikes.

Nature-appreciation activities can include virtually anything—nature-themed scavenger hunts, taking turns leading one another along a trail while blindfolded, or selecting natural objects along the way for use as clothing or play accessories. Such objects might include sticks for use as walking canes, tall grass stems as headdresses, or pinecones as baseballs.

Games can include verbal exercises like Progressive Storytelling, Twenty Questions, and I Spy, or physical activities such as Hide-and-Seek, or Relay (passing a stick backward from one hiker to another like runners passing a baton).

Logan and I entertained ourselves on one high-country hike with a game we developed ourselves. Every few yards, Logan would run ahead of me up the trail and lie down in a patch of skunk cabbage while I waited with my eyes closed. When he was hidden, I headed up the trail looking for him while muttering, "Fee, fie, foe, fum. I smell the blood of an Englishman." If I passed Logan without spotting him—which, no surprise, happened nearly every time—he crept up the trail behind me and startled me with a yell and a leap on my back. We repeated this over and over again.

Although I didn't do as much hiking that day as I might have, I had more fun leapfrogging slowly along the trail with Logan than I've had on any other dayhike I can remember.

> We banished the term "dayhike" from our parenting lexicon as quickly as we had the term "errand."

"Extreme" Dayhiking

One sunny, late-spring morning, Sue and I convinced Taylor and Logan to head out with us for a dayhike to the ruins of an abandoned silver mine high above timberline in the mountains north of Durango. We piqued the boys' interest by admitting the truth: We weren't sure we'd be able to make it to the mine because it was still early in the season, and we didn't know whether the route was clear or covered in snow.

We parked where the remains of a midwinter avalanche covered the road a mile before the trailhead. The boys led us over the avalanche debris and on to the end of the road. From there, Sue, the boys, and I had a great time simply trying to follow the trail, which required us to make our way over and around a series of steep snow-fields that clung to depressions in the mountainside.

Snow clogged the trail where it switchbacked through a north-facing cliff band a half mile from the mine. We left the trail and worked our way to a stretch of the cliff that faced the sun. There, the rock face was free of snow, but not of snowmelt. Spotting one another, we climbed from slippery ledge to slippery ledge until we topped the face.

Above the cliff, we ran into a four-person crew setting the course for a Red Bull Adventure Race scheduled to pass along the trail in a few days. The leader of the course crew told the boys how impressed he was that they'd made it so far up the trail. The day before, he said, his crew had been stopped by the cliff band the boys had just climbed. He'd brought his crew in via a less arduous route today, he explained, carrying shovels to dig out the snow covering the trail through the band of cliffs.

Energized by the crew leader's praise, the boys took off ahead of Sue and me across the flat

How to Make Your Dayhike Fun for the Family

1. Call it **anything but "hiking."** Say you're taking your kids exploring, climbing, bouldering, or mountaineering—and be sure to include elements of those in your hike.

2. **Include your kids** in preparations. Have them study maps, help prepare food for the adventure, and pack their own daypacks. Such activities will get them excited about the trip.

3. Always **have a goal** so your kids will know what they're setting out to accomplish. A lake, creek, cliff face, giant boulder, or the top of something—a mountain, hill, ridge, or bluff—all work well.

4. Let your **kids lead the way**. Let them be "boss" and set the pace.

5. Use any means available to **distract your kids** from the task of placing one foot in front of the other:

   ■ Tell **stories** and play **games**.

   ■ Supply them with **cameras** to use along the way.

   ■ Have your kids tie **stuffed animals** to their packs and act as tour guides and caretakers for their animals.

   ■ Allow your kids to carry their own **treats**, and assign them the task of deciding when to eat their treats. This will keep their minds surprisingly busy trying to determine whether to eat their favorite piece of candy at a particular trail junction or to save it until after lunch.

   ■ Have everyone **predict when you'll arrive** at your goal. Keep close track of distance traveled and time elapsed as the hike progresses. When you reach your goal, the person whose guess is closest to your arrival time wins an extra hunk of chocolate.

6. Do anything to **get your kids started**: crack jokes, sing songs, talk about future birthday parties. Once inertia is overcome, they'll generally settle in and have a great time.

7. **Experiment with activities** in the outdoors such as geocaching, orienteering, and trail running that equate to dayhiking for you, but are fun for your kids.

8. As your kids grow older, **choose dayhikes that challenge them** and you alike. Go "extreme" dayhiking.

snowfields that lay between the cliff and the abandoned mine.

The challenge of trying to reach the mine through the snow that day made what really was nothing more than a simple dayhike into a terrific family adventure. This sort of "extreme" dayhiking with your kids can include virtually anything of your choosing that makes a challenge of what otherwise would be a normal hike. Other forms of "extreme" dayhiking include hiking off trail to a high point, traversing a ridgeline end to end, tracking game or following a game trail as far as possible, or (one of my favorites) attempting to follow a water course to its source.

Possibilities

NATURE GAMES AND ACTIVITIES

The number of games and activities you can play with your youngsters while you dayhike with them is limited only by your imagination. To get your imagination cooking, visit www.sharingnature.com, the website of the Sharing Nature Foundation. The Sharing Nature Foundation was founded by naturalist and writer Joseph Cornell, author of *Sharing Nature With Children* (Dawn Publications 1998) and Sharing *Nature With Children II* (Dawn Publications 1998).

> The number of games and activities you can play with your youngsters while you dayhike with them is limited only by your imagination.

Sharing Nature With Children was first published in 1978. Since then, it has been translated into 19 languages. It is now considered the seminal work in the field of nature education. An updated edition of the book is available today.

On the foundation's website and in his books, Cornell describes a number of games and activities you can use to ensure you and your kids have fun on your dayhikes together. In particular, Cornell talks about how important it is for parents to bring a sense of wonder to all the outdoor activities they pursue with their children. More than anything else, Cornell says, it is that sense of wonder, willingly shared by parents, that draws children to the outdoor world and leads to their lifelong appreciation of it—and the simple act of tramping along a trail.

Geocaching Gear Tip

If you want to try geocaching a time or two without buying a GPS unit, consider renting a unit from Lower Gear (www.lowergear.com), which will ship the devices anywhere in the country. Otherwise, basic GPS units—all you need for geocaching—are available for less than $100.

GEOCACHING

Geocaching offers a tremendous opportunity for you to take your kids dayhiking without any worries your kids will complain that you're actually taking them on a forced march. Why? Because your kids won't see what they're

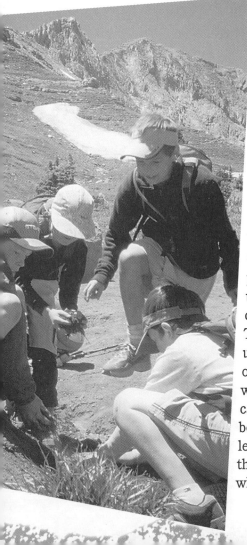

doing as dayhiking. Rather, they'll be on a treasure hunt. Moreover, in perfectly understandable little-kid terms, geocaching will introduce your youngsters to the fun and challenge of setting out to achieve a goal in the outdoors.

Essentially, geocaching is treasure hunting for big and little kids alike. Geocachers use global positioning system (GPS) units to locate hidden caches—usually Tupperware containers—using coordinates posted on the internet at www.geocaching.com. A cache generally holds a log book and small "treasures" left by the person who hid the container and those who since have found it.

Cache finders who wish to take a treasure from a cache are encouraged to leave a treasure in return.

The sport was born in 2000, when GPS use was opened to the general public. Since then, geocaching has boomed along with the internet and the availability of affordable GPS units (see "Geocaching Gear Tip," page 113). These days, www.geocaching.com tracks more than 100,000 active caches in more than 200 countries. Nearly 100,000 cache finds are logged at the geocaching website each week.

To choose an appropriate geocaching dayhike, simply go to the website, enter the location area that interests you, and surf potential cache sites to find one that suits your desired location, distance, and difficulty level. As you check out hike possibilities, you'll note that many caches are hidden in or near cities and towns. Plenty more, however, are located along trails in city, county, state, and national open spaces, parks, and forests—great places for dayhikes.

Of course, you can always set up your own geocaching adventure by hiding your own cache and noting its location coordinates in advance, then working with your kids to hike to and discover the cache. Another variation could be leading your kids on a wilderness scavenger hunt.

ORIENTEERING

The US Orienteering Federation defines orienteering as "an outdoor sport using maps and compasses to find one's way." Much like geocaching, orienteering offers you the opportunity to take your kids on a mentally engaging dayhike that is more fun than a simple walk through the woods.

The sport involves hiking or running (or even skiing, canoeing, or mountain biking) to a series of points on a

Compass and Map 101

Most orienteers prefer special compasses that attach to the thumb so they can easily check their direction of travel as they race through the woods. For an "orienteering" dayhike with your kids, however, any compass will do.

The key point to remember is that the red end of the compass needle always points northward toward the earth's magnetic north pole (as long as no metal or magnetic objects are near the compass). Using that critical piece of information, you'll be able to use any map for your dayhike—even one you've drawn yourself—to do some rough reckoning with your kids at the outset and along the course of your route.

How to do so? Simply lay the map on the ground or hold it before you, then lay your compass on it. Next, "orient" the map by turning the map beneath the compass until the map's north and the northward-pointing needle of the compass are aligned. Now take a general reckoning of the direction you wish to head with your kids and set off.

Your kids may want to lead the way while holding compasses in their hands. Rather than staring down at their compasses, they'll best be able to head in the correct direction if they choose points in the distance such as a large tree to walk toward. Don't worry much about whether they head in the "right" direction, though. Remember, the idea is to have a fun dayhike with your kids, not to frustrate them by trying to turn them into instant orienteers.

In fact, rather than orienteering with your kids, you might even choose to use a compass, colored pencils, and blank sheets of paper to do just the opposite of orienteering—that is, to roughly reckon your direction and distance as you hike, then team up with your kids to draw up a map of your route as you go.

For clear, detailed lessons on reading a compass and map, along with simple information you can pass on to your kids, go to www.learn-orienteering.org.

map as quickly as possible. The points, located at distinct features such as stream junctions or hilltops, are marked with flags as well as punches participants use to prove they've been there. Highly detailed maps that include features such as trees and boulders are used by those who are serious about orienteering. For dayhike orienteering with kids, any map will do, even one you've drawn yourself. Taking your youngster orienteering is simple. Here's how to do it:

1. Take them out for a dayhike of your choosing.

2. Bring along a topo map and compass.

3. Use it (or pretend to use it) along the way to "make sure you're not lost."

The result? You and your kids will have a terrific hike together—except that, as far as your kids are concerned, they'll have spent the hours of the hike "orienteering."

The same trick won't work twice, however. If you want to take your kids on another dayhike by going "orienteering," you'll need to up the ante a bit. For help in doing so, spend a few minutes at the US Orienteering Federation website (www.us.orienteering.org).

The site describes the federation's Little Troll program (keywords: Juniors or Youngsters). The site also details the federation's extensive race schedule, which includes more than 600 competitive meets across the country each year.

Further orienteering dayhikes with your kids can involve timed events along orienteering courses you plot on a map—courses that just happen to follow the dayhike routes you wish to take. There's no need to set a route in advance to pull this off. Simply choose a couple of points such as stream crossings or ridgetops on a topo map along a route you'd like to hike with your children. Then help your kids predict how long it'll take to reach each point. Keep careful time as you hike the route. Your kids will enjoy the anticipation of learning how close their predictions turn out to be—and you'll enjoy a fine dayhike with them.

TRAIL RUNNING

If you're a runner (or wish you were), you can take your kids trail running as a way to spice up a dayhike. There's no magic here. Just put on some good running shoes (see box), drive to the trailhead of your choosing, and set off. Depending on the ages of your children, they'll either run your socks off, or you'll spend your time on the trail with them running now and then but mostly hiking. Either way, you'll have accomplished what you set out for, and you'll

Healthy Feet

If your kids get serious about trail running, one piece of essential equipment is a pair of good-quality trail running shoes. Without them, you may compromise the long-term health of your children's growing feet. New Balance (www.newbalance.com) makes trail running shoes in children's sizes that work well for any of the forms of dayhiking discussed in this chapter.

have introduced them to an adventure sport that is growing steadily across the country.

Good trails for trail running are those that are generally flat or slightly uphill, making for a slightly downhill return to the trailhead. Obviously, smooth trails are better for running than rocky or root-bedeviled trails. In general, you'll be able to cover about as much ground on a "trail run" with your kids as you would during a dayhike. The distances you cover with your kids will be child- and trail-specific, but might range from a mile or so for youngsters to 3 or 4 miles for preadolescents.

Ultra trail runners are tackling unbelievable feats these days, including the Hardrock 100, a 48-hour, 100-mile trail run involving 66,000 vertical feet of elevation gain and descent near Silverton, Colorado, that is said to be the most difficult trail run on the ultra trail running circuit.

In addition to races such as the Hardrock, each year hard-core trail runners compete to break ultra long-distance records on famed trails such as the Mexico-to-Canada Pacific Crest Trail (2650 miles in 83 days), the John Muir Trail along California's Sierra Nevada spine (210 miles in just under four days), and the Denver-to-Durango Colorado Trail (487 miles in nine days).

Visit *Trail Runner* magazine's website (www.trailrunner-mag.com) for the latest from the world of trail running, including tips on trails you may wish to run or hike with your kids during any vacations you take around the country.

Trail running has grown so popular in recent years that trail-running guidebooks exist for various areas. Wilderness Press publishes

Trail Runner's Guide: San Diego and *Trail Runner's Guide: San Francisco Bay Area.*

SNOWSHOEING

The sport of snowshoeing has boomed in recent years with the advent of user-friendly snowshoe models for adults and child-specific models for kids. More than twice as many Americans snowshoe regularly these days as did just a few years ago.

Snowshoeing represents a great opportunity to get your kids excited about what is, essentially, a winter dayhike. Your kids will love the idea of heading out into the woods in the middle of winter.

Be aware, however, that actually going snowshoeing with kids can be problematic. It's difficult enough to get kids to keep moving while dayhiking. Snowshoeing is even harder because of the many layers of clothing kids must deal with, not to mention those pesky snowshoes.

The most kid-friendly snowshoe excursions take place on fairly flat trails already broken by other snowshoers. Warm sunny days are, obviously, best.

Don't be surprised if, only a few minutes after leaving your car, your kids opt to abandon their snowshoes and instead tumble down a nearby hill rather than continue trudging awkwardly along the trail. You won't be disappointed if you think of snowshoeing with your kids as more of an adventurous play outing than an actual hike.

Be sure to keep the "play outing" idea in mind when you dress your kids for snowshoeing. Waterproof snow pants are critical if your kids (and you) are to have a good time.

Stop often to add to or subtract from your kids' clothing layers. Cold kids are unhappy kids, and kids who get hot and sweaty while they snowshoe are likely to become chilled as soon as they stop to roll and play in the snow.

Hand warmers (available at outdoor and department stores) make great additions to youngsters' pockets during snowshoe excursions.

All snowshoe manufacturers make kid-size models, all of which essentially are small versions of each manufacturer's adult designs, and all of which function perfectly well. In addition, rental snowshoes are available virtually anywhere there's deep snow and a network of backcountry trails.

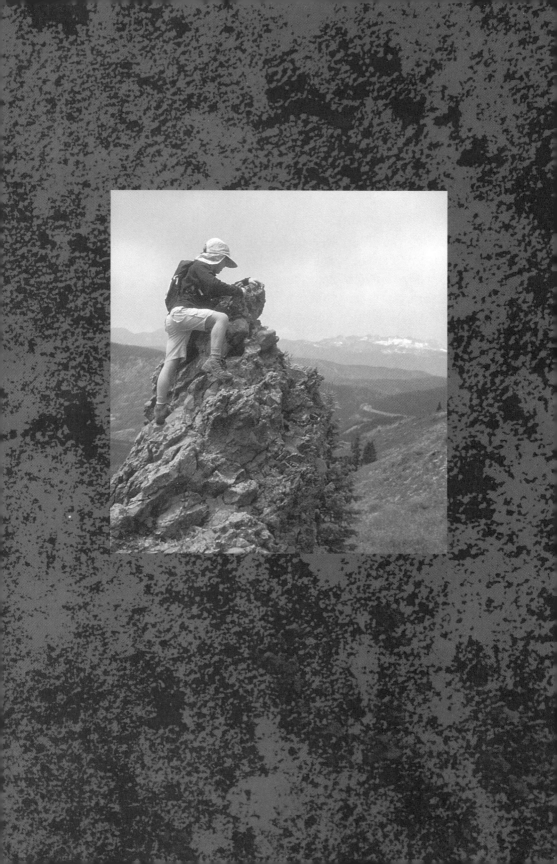

12 Peak Bagging

O ther than dayhiking, peak bagging is the simplest and most straightforward outdoor sport you can tackle with your kids.

The great thing about peak bagging with kids when they're very young is that just about anything will do. Climbs of concrete walls and decorative boulders beside supermarket parking lots will be major accomplishments to your kids as toddlers. With you as spotter, repeated ascents of the ladder up a playground slide—and taking in the view from way up there with big round eyes—will be plenty extreme for them.

Within a year or two of those toddler months, more realistic peak bagging with your kids is possible, as long as you continue to use the term loosely. Hills, low ridges, the high banks of creeks, anything *up* is a peak waiting to be bagged.

Such experiences will take your children to the age of 4 or 5, when they'll be ready for true peak bagging, provided you choose your peaks with care.

Choosing the Perfect Peak

Not long ago, Sammy, the 4-year-old daughter of friends, successfully climbed 14,150-foot Mt. Sneffels, namesake and high point of the Sneffels Range in west-central Colorado. Sneffels is a Class 2 climb (see "The Yosemite Decimal System," page 123).

It is also one of 54 peaks in Colorado that top out at more than 14,000 feet. The guidebook *Colorado's Fourteeners* (Fulcrum Publishing 1999) refers to the demanding route up the peak's south slopes as "a good route for someone who has climbed all the easy fourteeners and wants a taste of what the harder ones are like."

How was 4-year-old Sammy able to do the climb? The same as anybody else, her father says: One step at a time. The final summit push on Sneffels consists of a steep couloir filled with knee-high rocks requiring nimble footwork by adults. Those same rocks came up to Sammy's waist. "She just hoisted herself up on each one and kept going," her father says.

The Basics

■ When your kids are young, just about anything *up* is a peak waiting to be bagged. If you choose the right mountains, your kids will be capable of real mountain climbing by kindergarten age.

■ As they grow older, your kids will succeed at amazing feats of mountain climbing—provided you give them the opportunity as well as the encouragement they need.

■ More than just about any other sport, you must be subservient to what the weather dictates in order to keep your kids safe when mountain climbing with them.

Sammy's feat sounds impressive, and it was. But it also was well thought out by her parents. Of Colorado's fourteeners, Sneffels is one of the most accessible. The four-wheel-drive road to its base ends only a mile and a half from—and only 1800 vertical feet below—the mountain's summit.

Sammy didn't have to accomplish a lengthy approach hike to the peak. She simply had to step out of the car and start climbing—something virtually all 4-year-olds are good at. When you look for the perfect peak to climb with your kids, you'll want to keep the same sort of information in mind that Sammy's parents considered. It's better to choose a peak with a road to its base than one with a lengthy approach hike. And it's better to choose a peak you're sure you and your kids can handle.

Sammy's parents, experienced climbers, were comfortable escorting their young daughter up Sneffels' steep summit couloir. If you've not done much climbing yourself, you'll be best off starting with Class 1 climbs.

Note also that Class 2 climbs, in particular, are prone to a great deal of variation in difficulty level. In addition to the Class 2 rating, some guidebooks further describe those climbs as easy, medium, or difficult. You'll likely want to start off on the easier end of the Class 2 scale.

The Yosemite Decimal System

The Yosemite Decimal System has been used for more than 75 years to rate the difficulty level of various mountain climbs. Each climb is rated by its hardest portion, or crux.

Class 1 denotes easy climbing, generally on an established trail, all the way to the summit.

Class 2 denotes more difficult climbing, generally off trail. Some placing of hands may be necessary for balance.

Class 3 routes are steep and may entail a great deal of exposure. They require scrambling and using hands to make the ascent.

Class 4 routes are true climbing routes. They often require the use of ropes because falls can be fatal.

Class 5 denotes technical climbing that involves the use of ropes and belaying.

Unfortunately, no guidebooks cover the best peaks to climb with kids. Instead, you'll be faced with researching on your own any regions and peaks that interest you. It's best to start with some general climbing guidebooks to various areas, along with calls or visits to local outdoor stores in those areas.

Mountains present real dangers in the form of lightning and severe storms. More than perhaps any other activity in this book, you'll want to keep that fact in mind and be willing to turn around short of the summit should the weather dictate that you do so.

PRESIDENTIAL CLIMB

Sue and I went through a decision-making process similar to that of Sammy's parents when we chose a climb as part of a trip we took to the Northeast when Logan was 7.

Before we flew east, we had no idea which peak we would climb during our trip. We knew only that we wanted to get a taste of the Appalachians with our boys during the trip, and attempting to bag a peak seemed a logical way to do that.

We read up on various peaks while we dayhiked, fly-fished, and blueberry picked our way through Vermont and New Hampshire. We quickly settled on the Presidential Range of New Hampshire's White Mountains, the highest peaks in the East, for the challenge they presented and the above-tree-level views their summits afforded.

But which of the Presidentials to climb? The highest, 6288-foot Mt. Washington, with its paved road and cog railway to a summit cluttered with parking lots and a restaurant, gift shop, observatory, and other buildings, didn't interest us.

But the next peak north of Washington and the third highest in the range, 5718-foot Mt. Jefferson, did. Could 7-year-old Logan climb Jefferson? We weren't sure. (Though we knew we could always turn back if necessary.)

A map revealed that the easiest route up the mountain was via Jefferson's Caps Ridge on the mountain's west side. We liked the fact that the Caps Ridge Trail left Jefferson Notch Road at 3008 feet above sea level, the highest trailhead in the Presidential Range. That meant we had to climb only 2700 vertical feet over the course of 2.5 miles along the peak's west ridge to the summit. (I use the term "only," but 2700 feet is still half a mile of vertical gain.)

We got a good taste of the difference between New England climbing and Rocky Mountain climbing as soon as we set off. The trail plunged from the road into a buggy, boggy tangle of thick forest, through which the sun barely penetrated. High humidity made the air in the forest thick, and we were sweating heavily within minutes. The moist environment beneath the forest canopy meant the rocks and roots that comprised most of the trail were treacherously slick underfoot.

After a long mile, the trail broke free of the trees and switchbacked up the ridge proper. Here, the heat gave way to a chilly breeze. We layered up and kept moving. To the north across a broad valley, the steam-powered cog train spit thick black smoke into the air as it chuffed up Mt. Washington.

We made the summit of Jefferson long after the train made the summit of Washington, but the view was more rewarding than it would have been if we had taken the train. The view was also far different from the ones we were accustomed to in the Rockies. Rather than distant views of jagged peaks, we were greeted with pleasant views of rolling greenery stretching into the hazy distance.

The climb was plenty extreme for 7-year-old Logan, who beamed with pride at successfully summiting the peak with his older brother. When Sue and I reached the top a few minutes behind him, he proudly showed us the summit register and set about signing his name in it.

The benefit of the climb was the same as for every peak we climb with our boys: We were able to attempt—and, in this case, pull off—a challenging outdoor adventure with Taylor and Logan that required a minimum of equipment and fuss. All we needed was dayhiking gear and a day of

Attempting to bag a peak seemed a logical way to get a taste of the Appalachians with our boys.

our vacation. In return, we experienced mountains far different than those that surround our Colorado home. That experience became the high point, literally and figuratively, of our trip to the Northeast.

It's interesting to note that, like 4-year-old Sammy, Logan had no specific experience that enabled him to complete the Jefferson climb. He had done plenty of dayhiking and other outdoor sports before attempting Jefferson, but the climb itself required nothing more of Logan than stamina and placing one foot in front of the other.

Hand Protection

Youngsters tend to slip and fall regularly on steep slopes. They often end up with owies when they put out their hands to catch themselves.

You can minimize this problem by holding your kids' hands as much as possible when you're negotiating steep stretches with them. It's impossible to hold your kids' hands all the time, though. To further minimize the scrapes your youngsters may suffer, have them wear lightweight mittens to protect their sensitive palms when they fall, even on warm days.

He completed what was a tough climb for him not because he'd worked his way up to it, but because the climb was one Sue and I, as experienced climbers, were comfortable leading him on, and because we encouraged him and praised his progress all along the way.

Climbing isn't easy for youngsters. More than once on the way up Jefferson, Logan asked about the possibility of turning around. Your kids likely will ask the same of you when you're climbing a peak with them. Despite that reality, climbing is worthwhile for youngsters because of the tremendous sense of accomplishment they get from summiting a mountain. Today Logan continues to swell with pride when he sees the snapshot Sue took of him with Taylor atop Jefferson, and I have no doubt that pride is something that transfers directly into other endeavors Logan takes on—such as, most recently, trying out for a part in a local theater production.

Possibilities

Many people consider true peak bagging to have as a goal the summiting of as many peaks on a given list as possible—the 48 4000-foot peaks in New Hampshire, for example, or the 54 fourteeners in Colorado. In contrast, knocking off one peak of any definition from any list (or from no list at all) constitutes peak bagging as far as the family-oriented possibilities that follow are concerned.

FIFTY HIGH POINTS

I vividly remember, as a 9-year-old in Ohio, walking the grassy slope to the top of Campbell Hill, the highest point in the state. My "climb" to the "summit" of Ohio wasn't extreme. But it fired in my imagination the desire to climb high peaks, and when my family moved to the

mountains of Colorado a year later, I considered myself the luckiest kid in the world.

Many of the highest points in the 50 states aren't exactly high. (For example, the highest physical point in Illinois, if you include manmade objects, is the top of the Sears Tower in downtown Chicago.) Most are near, and many are topped by, roads. Still, seeking out and "climbing" the highest point in your state is a good way to introduce peak bagging to your kids. From there, the sky literally is the limit.

The Highpointers Club is dedicated to tracking those who have climbed the high points in all 50 states, and to maintaining access to the 50 high points, many of which are on private property. Visit the club's website at www.highpointers.org for detailed directions to the high point in your state.

INCLUDE PEAK BAGGING DAYS IN YOUR VACATIONS

There's no better way to get an overview of an area you're visiting than to climb high and look down at it.

For your kids, a peak bagging day generally will beat a hiking day because setting out to summit a hill or bluff or mountain will provide them with a clear goal. You'll do plenty of encouraging along the way to get them to achieve that goal, but they'll be incredibly proud when they do.

Unless you're planning a vacation to Florida, the possibilities are endless for finding "peaks" to "bag." Here are a few options:

■ Visiting San Francisco? Schedule a day to head north across the Golden Gate Bridge and climb Mt. Tamalpais (called Mt. Tam by locals: www.mttam.net) in Mt. Tamalpais State Park. Summiting the 2571-foot peak (chockablock with people on sunny weekend days) requires either a stroll from a nearby parking lot or a longer climb up a trail from a lower road. On clear days, the view of San Francisco and the rest of the Bay Area from the top of the mountain is fantastic.

■ Visiting Gettysburg National Military Park in southeastern Pennsylvania? Don't simply follow the driving route through the battlegrounds. Be sure to climb with your kids to the top of rocky Devil's Den (www.nps.gov/gett), site of some of the Battle of Gettysburg's fiercest fighting as Union soldiers sought to hold the high point against the Confederate Army's advance.

■ Visiting Phoenix? Hike up 2608-foot Piestewa Peak (www-phoenix.gov/parks; keyword: Piestewa) in Phoenix Mountains Park for a panoramic view of the Phoenix metropolitan area.

■ In Denver, check out two 14,000-foot peaks, Grays and Torreys, which are less than an hour's drive west of the city on I-70. The peaks, respectively the 9th and 11th highest in the state, constitute a fine, though demanding, day climb, and are justifiably crowded on summer weekends.

Youngsters will do well with just the goal of summiting Grays Peak. Older kids may have the stamina to cross the ridge that connects Grays and Torreys and summit Torreys as well. If you and your kids climb the pair of fourteeners early in the season, you'll be able to glissade the snow slope that clings to the face of the connecting ridge until late June most years. See www.14ers.com for route descriptions.

Colorado Fourteener pins (www.toppeak.com), available for each of Colorado's 14,000-foot peaks, make great rewards for climbs of Grays, Torreys, or any of the state's 52 other fourteeners.

SETTING YOUR SIGHTS ON SPECIFIC PEAKS

As your children grow older, you can build a vacation around peaks you want to climb rather than finding a high point to climb as part of a vacation you've already planned. Doing so will mean heading to the mountains.

There's no better way to get an overview of an area you're visiting than to climb high and look down at it.

Again, the possibilities are endless. To help narrow them down, try browsing the website www.peakbaggers.com. Among the countless possibilities are:

■ Mt. Sneffels (Colorado): A three-hour drive south of Grand Junction, this peak should not be taken lightly. It's true that 4-year-old Sammy climbed the peak. But it's also true that the high-altitude climb of Sneffels will be plenty arduous for you and your kids if you live at or near sea level. In addition, the final portion of the climb involves exposed, hand-over-hand maneuvering. The website www.14ers.com has a good description, with photos, of the route up Mt. Sneffels' south slopes.

■ Mt. Jefferson (New Hampshire): Exercise extreme caution on Mt. Jefferson, which is a three-hour drive from Boston. Storms that quickly gather over the Presidential Range kill hikers and climbers every year. With kids it'll be especially important for you to turn back at the earliest hint of bad weather. Note that although Logan managed the Caps Ridge Trail without difficulty at age 7, the website www.peakbaggers.com calls the trail "steep and very rugged," and "best avoided by novice hikers." For information on Mt. Jefferson, visit www.fs.fed.us (keywords: White Mountain).

■ Springer Mountain (Georgia): Just two hours from Atlanta, Springer Mountain offers an easy 2-mile hike from Forest Service Road 42 to the top at 3820 feet. Springer Mountain is considered by Appalachian Trail devotees as almost holy ground because the trail leads to the summit plaque that marks the southern terminus/starting point of the 2100-mile Appalachian Trail.

Hiking to the top of Springer Mountain with your kids will introduce them to the idea of thru-hiking on long-distance trails, especially if you time your summit-bound hike for late March or early April, when most Appalachian Trail thru-hikers set off from the mountain, headed for Maine. Though it isn't officially part of the Appalachian Trail, the trail to the top of Springer is blazed with the well-known white rectangles that mark the entire route of the Appalachian Trail.

Visit www.georgiatrails.com for detailed information on the hike/climb.

■ Mt. St. Helens (Washington): Just an hour's drive from Portland, Oregon, in southwestern Washington, 8365-foot Mt. St. Helens will provide your kids with a good introduction to the idea of mountaineering in the Northwest.

When volcanic activity hasn't closed the mountain, which blew its top in 1980 and is still an active volcano, the Forest Service issues 100 permits each day from April through October. The cost is $15 per person to those who wish to climb to the volcano's crater. The easiest route up the volcano isn't exactly easy; it's 5 miles and 4500 vertical feet to the rim via the Monitor Ridge route. The trail up the ridge is suitable for older children. It's long and steep but not technically demanding.

Visit www.fs.fed.us/gpnf for more information.

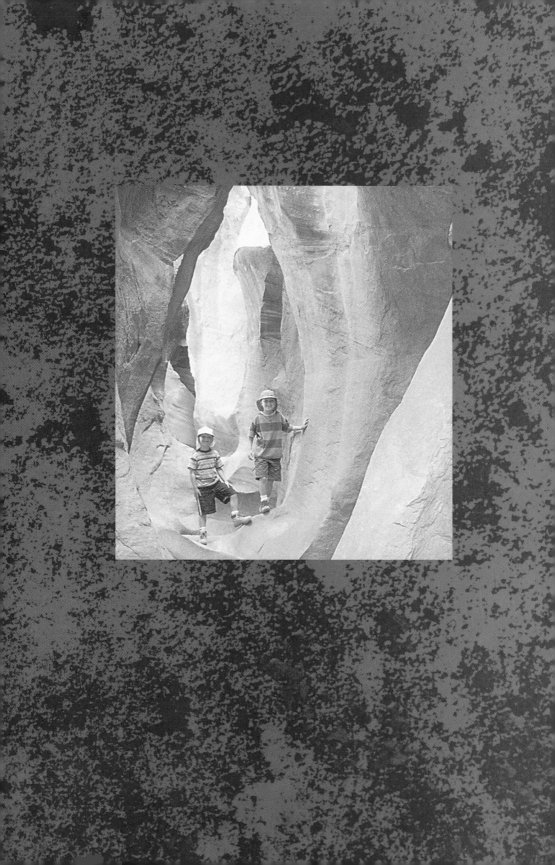

13 Canyoneering

The Zion Adventure Company, which leads and out-fits trips into the sandstone slot canyons of Zion National Park, calls canyoneering "the most fun you can have as a grown-up." I'd amend that to call canyoneering "the most fun you can have with your kids."

Canyoneering is the opposite of peak bagging. It is no more and no less than the simple act of traveling through canyons.

At its least extreme, canyoneering is a straightforward walk through a dry, narrow, flat-bottomed canyon—a nice alternative to a trail-based dayhike with your kids. At the other end of the spectrum, canyoneering is an ultra-extreme outdoor sport involving all manner of technical gear and expertise in order to traverse deep, water-filled slot canyons featuring waterfalls, pools, overhangs, cliffs, drop-offs, and rapids.

Today, canyoneering is a booming sport in the US, and it long has been popular in Europe and other parts of the world (where it is known as "canyoning"). Most important for you, canyoneering presents unlimited potential for having fun in the outdoors with your kids.

The only very real drawback to canyoneering is that it is site specific. Unlike dayhiking, which can be done any-where in the outdoors, canyoneering requires a canyon. Though explorable canyons exist in many parts of the US, the primary canyoneering region of the country is the

Colorado Plateau, an expanse of many-layered sandstone straddling the Arizona/Utah border. The massive plateau's name is derived from the fact that the sandstone of the plateau is cut by countless slot canyons that flow, eventually, to the Colorado River.

No doubt you've seen beauty shots in outdoor magazines of canyoneers gazing from the floors of deep canyons at incredible walls of red and ocher sandstone lit by shafts of sunlight streaming down from above. Virtually all such pictures were taken in the Colorado Plateau slot canyons of southern Utah and northern Arizona.

Starting Easy

When your kids are youngsters, you can get away with calling just about any water drainage a "canyon" and just about any hike along a water course "canyoneering." Soon enough, however, if you talk up the idea of going canyoneering with your kids, they're going to expect the real thing. How to pull that off?

Schedule a day or two of canyoneering—or a canyoneering-oriented backpacking trip—with your kids as part of a family vacation to the Southwest. A lifetime's worth of canyons await you within an easy rental car's drive of Las Vegas, Phoenix, Albuquerque, Denver, or Salt Lake City.

Sue and I began canyoneering with our boys the spring after Logan turned 6. That April, we pulled our boys out of school for a week and took off with them for nine days of exploring the scads of sandstone slot canyons in south-central Utah's huge Grand Staircase-Escalante National Monument. In our previous life as a child-free couple, Sue and I had hiked and explored many of the slots in the region on our own. Now we were anxious to try canyoneering with our boys.

The first thing we did on our visit to the monument was head east out of the tiny town of Escalante on the Hole-in-the-Rock Road to the trailhead for Peek-a-Boo, Spooky, and Brimstone canyons, famous side-by-side slots we'd purposefully avoided in the years before we had children because we knew how much fun it would be to explore them with kids.

There may be no better playground for children, manmade or otherwise, than the three slots we explored that day. Peek-a-Boo, Spooky, and Brimstone are easy-to-explore slot canyons, so narrow you have to turn sideways to make your way through them. Their flat, sandy floors are simple for youngsters to navigate, and the sun-streaked walls provide endless beauty, at times as curvaceous as a snow cornice, at others as linear as if cleaved by a butcher knife.

The Basics

- A walk through just about any depression in the earth can constitute an exciting "canyoneering" adventure when your kids are little.

- Slot-canyon adventures range from giggle-filled walks through tight passages to guided rope-and-rappel tours of deep sandstone fissures.

- For true slot-canyon hiking with your kids, you'll need to head to the Colorado Plateau region where Utah and Arizona meet.

- As your kids get older, you can combine canyoneering with family backpacking trips.

Images best describe the fun Sue and I had with Taylor and Logan that day: leaving the hot desert day behind and diving into the cool, dusky half-light of each canyon; marveling at the play of sunlight filtering down from narrow cracks of blue sky high overhead; worrying as Taylor and Logan crawled deeper into the slots than Sue's and my larger bodies would allow, then relief as they squeezed their way back to us inch by squealing-with-excitement inch.

When you get right down to it, our day of canyoneering with Taylor and Logan consisted of nothing more than slithering our way between tight walls of sandstone—not overly extreme as extreme sports go. But our day was, in a word, phenomenal.

In the years since, Sue and I have hiked and explored many other canyons with Taylor and Logan, as dayhikes

135

and as multiday backpacking trips, and every one of our canyon-exploration experiences has been tremendously fun.

"Extreme" Canyoneering

Many canyoneers would sneer at the type of hike-and-explore canyoneering Sue and I have done with our boys. To true canyoneers, it ain't canyoneering unless it involves ropes; harnesses; drysuits; belay and ascension devices; the potential for entrapment, hypothermia, and/or drowning; and heinous rappels off overhangs and through waterfalls into dark, little-known depths.

Extreme canyoneering of that sort doesn't make for much of a family outing, but you couldn't tell that to Leo Lloyd. Lloyd is one of the top rope-rescue-course instructors in the country. When Lloyd's son Kendall was 10, Lloyd took him down Mystery Canyon in Zion National Park. Decked out in full canyoneering gear, Kendall dropped 2000 vertical feet down the canyon over a series of 11 rappels, most in the midst of waterfalls and into deep pools.

Canyoneering Footwear

If you'll be taking your kids into a canyon such as the Zion Narrows, which involves wading in water, logic might tell you to shoe your kids in strap-on water sandals.

But while strap-on sandals are great for most water sports, they're not good for slogging in creeks. For that, your children should wear above-the-ankle hiking boots to protect their feet and ankles from slippery underwater rock.

The only canyoneering-specific shoe in the world, a beefy neoprene strap-on appropriately named the Canyoneer, is made by Five.Ten (www.fiveten.com). The Canyoneer retails for around $100 and comes in women's sizes down to size 5, but it is not available in children's sizes. Canyoneers are available for rent from outfitters in the town of Springdale, Utah, at the mouth of Zion Canyon.

The final rappel out of Mystery Canyon drops 100 feet, in the middle of a waterfall, straight into the popular day-hiking section of the national park's Zion Canyon Narrows. When Kendall dropped from Mystery Canyon into the Narrows, his father reports, dayhikers stopped and gawked at him as if he'd just arrived from the moon.

Lloyd says he works at "making quality memories" for his kids of the sort Kendall took from the Mystery Canyon expedition. "I want to do things with my kids that they can really build on in their own lives," Lloyd says. "I want them to be comfortable with themselves when they're older, comfortable doing things they want to do—even if the things they do aren't what everyone else does."

> **When Kendall dropped from Mystery Canyon into the Narrows, dayhikers stopped and gawked at him as if he'd just arrived from the moon.**

To get ready for Mystery Canyon, Lloyd spent two weeks working with Kendall on his rope skills. In addition, the 10-year-old had rock climbed regularly with his father for several years. Even so, the canyoneering trip itself was highly structured for Kendall. "We always sent someone from our group of adults down before Kendall," says Lloyd, "and on the longer rappels I joined him on the rope."

The result was a safe yet incredibly extreme outing for a 10-year-old.

A canyoneering expedition of the type Kendall accomplished with his father in Mystery Canyon is beyond the realm of most families. However, one outfitter, Zion Adventure Company, regularly approximates extreme canyoneering in less arduous canyons in southwestern

Utah for families with children as young as 5. If you have the cash and you and your kids have the inclination, such an outfitted adventure (detailed on page 139) offers a terrific opportunity for your entire family to get a taste of extreme canyoneering.

Possibilities

ZION CANYON NARROWS

Located just two and a half hours from Las Vegas, the Zion Canyon Narrows, formed by the Virgin River in the heart of Zion National Park (www.nps.gov/zion) in southwestern Utah, is the most popular slot canyon hike on Earth—and a perfect way to introduce your kids to the fun and challenges of canyoneering. (Note: The hike into the Narrows is recommended for children 4 feet tall or taller, roughly ages 5 and up.)

A paved trail leads a mile into the Narrows. At the end of the trail, where the canyon walls tighten and the (normally) shallow Virgin River extends from canyon wall to canyon wall, you and your kids may simply step into the water and wade upstream. The farther you go, the more the 1000-foot walls of the canyon will close in around you.

As with all canyoneering excursions, you'll be able to hike the Narrows only when the river is low and free of flash-flood danger. (In dry southwestern Utah, that's most of the year.) Wading the Narrows is a cool—as in *not* warm—experience, even when the surrounding desert outside the canyon is egg-fry hot. Though canyoneers explore the Narrows year round, you'll want to stick to warmer months with your kids to ensure they have fun.

The Narrows is an in-and-out hike; you can walk upstream as far as you and your kids want before turning around and making your way out. Dayhikers are allowed to walk the river several miles without getting a permit from the park. (Because of the demanding nature of walking in the riverbed, your trip with your kids will be far shorter than that.)

Even more than with other outdoor adventures with kids, the key in the Narrows is to not overdo it. A greater percentage of your kids' bodies will be in the water while wading up the river. As a result, your kids will get colder and more tired more quickly than you will. It'll be up to you to carefully judge when your party should turn back.

Remember, simply making it a few bends beyond the end of the paved trail is a very real accomplishment for kids, provided you turn back early enough to ensure that the journey out of the Narrows is as fun as the journey in.

Outfitters in the town of Springdale at the mouth of Zion Canyon rent canyoneering footwear (see "Canyoneering Footwear," page 136), dry pants, and sturdy walking sticks for trips into the Narrows. On hot days, you might be able to get away without dry pants and canyoneering-specific footwear, but sturdy walking sticks—either rentals or collapsible trekking poles you've brought with you—are a must for everyone in your party.

ZION ADVENTURE COMPANY'S FAMILY ADVENTURE DAY

From March through November each year, Springdale, Utah-based Zion Adventure Company offers a Family Adventure Day for families with children ages 5 and up. The day is spent learning and applying the basics of technical canyoneering in one of Zion National Park's many slot canyons.

The day includes instruction in knot tying, anchor placement, belaying, and rappelling. Participants complete up to four rappels during a daylong slot-canyon descent. The rappels range from 20 to 100 feet.

The outfitter provides all gear necessary for the trip. All you need to bring is food, water, and, as the company's brochure puts it, "consensus"—that is, that this something all members of your family want to do. The day costs approximately $500 for a family of four. For more information about Zion Adventure Company, call 435-772-0990 or visit www.zionadventures.com.

PEEK-A-BOO, SPOOKY, AND BRIMSTONE CANYONS

As noted earlier in this chapter, these three short, tight slot canyons in south-central Utah may well be the most kid-friendly slots on the planet. The three canyons, which open onto the Dry Fork tributary of Coyote Gulch in the heart of Grand Staircase-Escalante National Monument, are easily explored in a day. They're located 25 miles down the graded Hole-in-the-Rock Road, which leaves Utah Hwy. 12 about 5 miles east of the town of Escalante. The parallel slots are a half mile from one another and less than a mile's hike from the side-road trailhead, which is accessible by rental car. The stunningly scenic drive to Escalante takes about five hours from either Las Vegas or Salt Lake City.

Be prepared for desert hiking conditions outside the slots and refreshing coolness in them.

Since the creation of Grand Staircase-Escalante National Monument in the late 1990s, the slot canyons of the Escalante River drainage have become increasingly popular, and none more so than Peek-a-Boo, Spooky, and Brimstone. If you and your kids want to avoid waiting your turn to slither inside the three slots, arrive at the trailhead early in the day. (An early arrival will avail you and your kids of the best time of day to hike in the desert—the early morning hours when winds are calm and temperatures cool.)

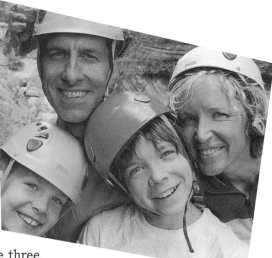

After your exploration of the three slots, be sure to stop off to play in Devil's Garden on your way back up the Hole-in-the-Rock Road. Devil's Garden is a compact group of sandstone sculptures, arches, and towers. No trails wind through the "garden." You and your kids are free to walk around and scramble up on the rock formations.

For detailed information on hiking Peek-a-Boo, Spooky, and Brimstone, go to www.canyoneeringusa.com/ utah/esca/drycoy.htm.

WATER HOLES CANYON

While Arizona's world-famous Antelope Canyon, known as the most photographed slot canyon on Earth, is a stunning slot canyon, visiting it is an expensive endeavor. Instead, you and your kids can enjoy exploring nearby Water Holes Canyon, a slot that lies 6 miles south of Page (a five-hour drive from Phoenix), perpendicular to US Hwy. 89.

You will have to pay a few dollars per person to visit the canyon, which lies on Navajo Reservation land, but you won't be faced with paying the big bucks required to visit Antelope, nor will you have to deal with Antelope's crowds. Instead, you'll be able to drop from the parking area straight into quiet, high-walled Water Holes, sections of which are nearly as beautiful as Antelope.

For a good description and photos of Water Holes and many other Colorado Plateau slot canyons, visit www.americansouthwest.net/slot_canyons.

BUCKSKIN GULCH

For a true wilderness-like slot canyon experience with your kids, try Arizona's Buckskin Gulch, a side canyon of the Paria River 30 miles west of Page, off Hwy. 89.

With 12 miles of continuous narrows, Buckskin Gulch is the longest slot canyon in the Southwest. Many canyoneering aficionados consider it the best overall slot canyon on Earth.

At first glance, Buckskin Gulch doesn't appear kid friendly because canyoneers who travel deep into Buckskin must wade through mud- and muck-filled pot-holes, sometimes waist deep, that remain full months after the canyon's periodic floods. For parents in the know, however, Buckskin Gulch provides a great canyoneering-with-kids experience. A low-walled side slot called Wire Pass, beautiful in its own right, provides easy access, after a 1.5-mile hike and a couple of simple down-climbs over chockstones, to a stunning stretch of Buckskin Gulch. This area lacks the potholes that make travel with little kids difficult.

> **For parents in the know, Buckskin Gulch provides a great canyoneering-with-kids experience.**

Like many of the Colorado Plateau's most easily accessible slots, Wire Pass/Buckskin Gulch is a popular destination. You won't be alone there, but your hike will be so breathtakingly beautiful—and so enjoyable for your kids—you'll barely notice the other hikers.

Note that to undertake this hike, your children should be capable of 5 miles or so of rugged, off-trail, canyon-bottom hiking—a little over 3 miles round trip to Buckskin

Gulch via Wire Pass, plus a couple of miles of exploration in Buckskin proper.

The Wire Pass Trailhead is an easy drive west from Page on Hwy. 89 and 8 miles south on a graded dirt road. For detailed information on Wire Pass and Buckskin Gulch, go to www.americansouthwest.net/slot_canyons.

OTHER CANYONS

If you're willing to broaden your definitions of slot canyon and canyoneering enough, many drainages across the country work well either as "canyoneering" dayhikes with young children or backpacking trips with older kids. Some of these include:

Fern Canyon: A perfect dayhike, five hours from San Francisco, is Fern Canyon in Prairie Creek Redwoods State Park on the northern California coast. Fern Canyon is a half-mile-long, 50- to 80-foot-deep box canyon gouged into coastal sediment by tiny Home Creek. Every square inch of the canyon's earthen walls is festooned with ferns, making a trip there akin to exploring a moist green fairyland.

To visit Fern Canyon with your kids, you'll walk from the end of a remote road on the coast of the Pacific Ocean north of Orick, California, for a mile to the canyon's mouth. From there, leave the beach to stroll up the short canyon, leaping meandering Home Creek as necessary.

For more information, call Prairie Redwoods State Park at 707-464-6101 or visit www.redwoodvisitor.org (keywords: Fern Canyon).

143

Aravaipa Canyon: This canyon-oriented backpacking trip is located far south of the sandstone slot canyons of the Colorado Plateau in the Sonoran Desert region of southern Arizona. The downstream mouth of Aravaipa Canyon, located northeast of Tucson, is accessible by passenger cars; the upstream end requires high-clearance vehicles for access.

The magic of the canyon lies with Aravaipa Creek, which arises out of nowhere to run for a few miles, clear and cool, through an otherwise inhospitable desert. Water that runs beneath the surface of the upper Aravaipa drainage is forced above the ground by underlying rock where the walls of the canyon close together. For 11 miles thereafter, the creek runs between stands of saguaro and prickly pear cactus.

Then, where the canyon walls again widen, the creek disappears underground once more. Where it appears above ground, the creek is a narrow, meandering oasis for all manner of desert life, from javelina and desert bighorn sheep to scorpion, quail, and endangered, frog-eating black hawks, all of which Sue, Taylor, Logan, and I saw when we backpacked in the canyon.

Visiting Aravaipa requires calling weeks ahead for a permit. You'll spend much of your time wading in Aravaipa Creek itself, as no maintained trail exists in the canyon.

You may either dayhike or backpack in the canyon. Both are popular. Sue and I backpacked 1.5 miles into the canyon with Taylor and Logan and another family when our boys were 7 and 5. Our three-day trip was magical for the geographic dichotomy it offered—carefree water play in the creek with brutal desert only feet away.

For more information, call the Bureau of Land Management at 928-348-4400 or visit www.recreation.gov (keyword: Aravaipa).

More suggestions: Many magical water drainages such as Fern and Aravaipa exist across the country. Note, as further examples among many more: North Carolina's Panthertown Valley (as detailed on pages 165 and 166); Kings Canyon (www.nps.gov/seki) and Yosemite Valley (www.nps.gov/yose) in California; and Havasu Canyon and the incomparable waterfalls along Havasu Creek on the Havasupai Reservation at the western end of the Grand Canyon in central Arizona (www.havasupaitribe.com).

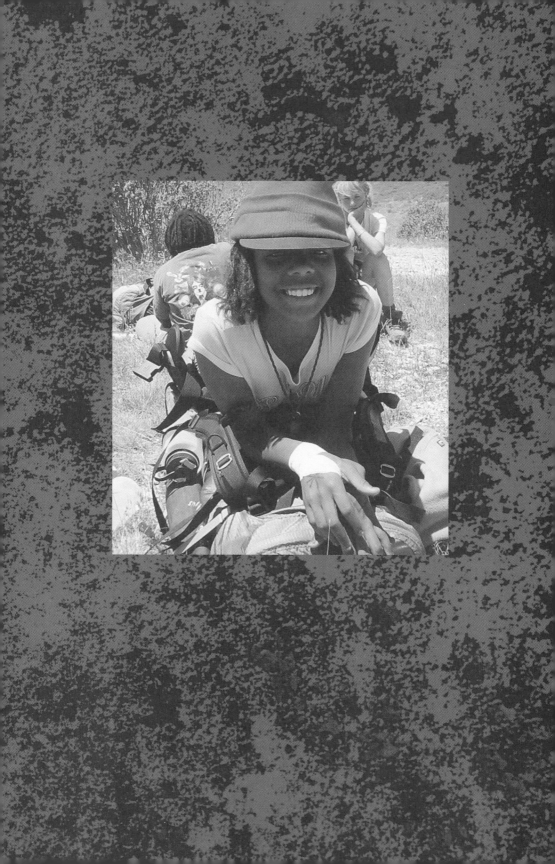

14 Backpacking

O ver the years, the number of Americans who choose to spend their leisure time backpacking has started to decline. According to the Outdoor Industry Association, the number of backpackers in the US has fallen by as much as 20 percent in recent years. The association reported that sales of backpacking gear have also gone down. If the coverage in *Backpacker* magazine is any indication, more people today are choosing shorter, quicker versions of outdoor hiking and adventuring.

To all of which, I say, "Great!"

Why should I be pleased fewer Americans are backpacking these days? Because the fewer people willing to peel themselves away from their jobs, television sets, video games, computer screens, and Super-Size meals to go backpacking, the more quiet trails there are for the rest of us to explore with our kids.

Self-centered? Maybe. True? Absolutely.

For a time during the backpacking boom of the 1970s and 1980s, many backpackers feared that their most beloved trails soon would be overrun. Instead, the nation's most popular backpacking locales such as the Grand Canyon and the John Muir Trail have seen a stabilization, and in some cases a decline, in user numbers. Officials in charge of controlling access to those locations have been able to institute and fine-tune permit and quota systems that protect popular trails from overuse while enabling reasonable access to those who wish to visit.

Thanks to these trends, it's fairly easy to get a permit to popular backpacking locations, as long as you plan ahead. Moreover, you can almost count on a crowd-free trip if you head out with your kids to any of the hundreds of terrific backpacking trails across the country that don't require permits.

Why Backpack?

Despite the drop in numbers of Americans backpacking these days, it's worth remembering that millions of Americans still backpack each year. They do so for the same reasons Sue and I enjoyed backpacking before we had kids and continue to enjoy it with Taylor and Logan today.

For adults, there's a lot to be said for getting away from cars, roads, houses, and the work-a-day world by going backpacking. For children, there's something magical about heading off into the woods and surviving for a few days on just the stuff you can carry on your back.

That sense of wonder and adventure stirs children's souls and excites them about the idea of backpacking. The actual doing of it, however, can be pretty hard on kids. But if you follow the tips in this chapter aimed at making backpacking a positive experience for your children, you'll find that backpacking with kids is actually a simple and straightforward process, and one your kids will thoroughly enjoy.

The Basics

- Your kids will find it truly magical to set off into the woods for two or three days and survive only on what you and they can carry.

- Being away from cars and television—and even from all the accoutrements of other, more extreme outdoor sports—for several days makes for unparalleled play and bonding opportunities between you and your kids.

- America's many hike-in campsites close to roads provide great opportunities for beginning backpacking trips for you and your kids.

- Thanks to a leveling in backpacker numbers, America's most famous backpacking trails are readily available to you and your kids as your kids grow older.

- Far more than on adult-only backpacking trips, the key to fun backpacking trips with kids is to go light, go light, go light.

First Tries

I worked at an REI store in the 1980s, during the heart of the backpacking boom. At the time, I was amazed when the store's manager and his wife backpacked to the bottom of the Grand Canyon and out with their five-month-old baby. The manager told me the trip had been tough but, ultimately, worthwhile.

Sue and I waited until Taylor was a toddler and Sue was five months pregnant with Logan before we tackled our first family backpacking trip. The trip, a 2-miler to the trickling creek that runs through Utah's redrock-walled Grand Gulch, wasn't easy.

I loaded a cavernous mountaineering pack with all of our gear and hiked to our campsite. In the meantime, Sue headed down the trail from the car holding Taylor's hand and wearing an empty child-carrier backpack. I dumped the big pack at the campsite and returned up the trail to Sue and Taylor. There, I loaded Taylor on my back in the child carrier and the three of us proceeded down the canyon to our camp. The next day, we repeated the process back to the car.

I'm the first to admit such a backpacking trip isn't for everybody. But Sue and I love to walk away from roads and cars and the hubbub of modern life as much as we can. That love of backpacking has only intensified as Taylor and Logan have grown older. In response, each year, Sue and I schedule several long weekends and at least one longer stretch for family backpacking trips.

Through all the backpacking we've done with Taylor and Logan over the last few years, Sue and I have developed a number of strategies that enable the four of us to enjoy backpacking as a family, which I outline below.

> For children, there's something magical about heading off into the woods and surviving for a few days on just the stuff you can carry on your back.

Take Crowded Trails

At first it may seem counterintuitive for me to recommend starting out on highly popular trails. The whole point of backpacking is to get away from it all—from cars, phones, TVs, and, most of all, those annoying fellow citizens of yours.

But backpacking is one of the more arduous and unavoidably boring (to youngsters) outdoor sports you can tackle with kids. Such a combination can turn a dream family backpacking trip into a nightmare.

Backpacking on a trail frequented by others when your kids are young gives your kids something to do—e.g. spot, make way for, and talk to all the other backpackers and hikers sharing the trail.

More important, heavily traveled trails offer built-in cheering sections for your kids. The other grown-ups you pass on the trail will "ooooh" and "aaahhh" all over your

Tips for Backpacking with Kids

- Start with popular trails.
- Team up with other families.
- Go lighter than you've ever gone before.
- Pick trips with good payoffs after short distances.
- Return to the car for a second load if necessary.
- Choose a destination near a ready-to-play-in water source.

pint-size packers. In response, your children will puff with pride and rocket up the trail.

Sue and I purposefully chose to hike the crowded Bright Angel Trail the first time we backpacked the Grand Canyon with Taylor and Logan. Bright Angel, which runs from the South Rim of the canyon to the confluence of the Colorado River and Bright Angel Creek in the bottom of the canyon, is the most popular trail in the Grand Canyon. Its upper couple of miles constitute one of the most heavily trodden trail sections in the country.

Logan, then 6, charged out of the canyon on Taylor's heels. He did so in large part, I'm convinced, because the many adult dayhikers and backpackers on the busy stretch of trail offered him a constant stream of encouraging comments all the way to the rim.

In addition to the encouragement your kids will receive, backpacking heavily used trails also will help make your kids aware of the fact that they are a part of a large community of people who appreciate the outdoors and enjoy exploring the wilds on foot.

When your kids grow older and are accustomed to the challenge and satisfaction of lugging a pack into the wilderness, you can search out little-used trails where only birds will serenade you.

JOIN FORCES

They say nothing is more powerful than peer pressure for teenagers. From what I've witnessed, the same is true for younger children (and adults, too, for that matter). When it comes to backpacking with your kids, it's worth taking peer pressure into account and teaming up with other families when you can.

Sue and I enjoy backpacking on our own with our boys, but we appreciate going out with other families as well. When we're on the trail with another family, we don't have to resort to the many tricks detailed in this book for keeping our boys' minds off the boring aspects of hiking along a trail. Taylor and Logan wouldn't dream of complaining when they're on the trail with other kids. Instead, they and the children of the families with whom we backpack cheerfully occupy themselves on the trail and in camp, while Sue and I are free to enjoy ourselves and the company of the other adults with whom we're hiking and camping.

GO LIGHT, GO LIGHT, GO LIGHT

Though every backpacking guidebook recommends going light, child-free adult backpackers can—and usually do—get away with bringing a few luxuries along on their trips. In the case of backpacking with kids, however, you must take this recommendation to heart.

There simply are too many necessities to bring when you go backpacking with your kids—the bulk of which you'll be responsible for carrying. Anything extraneous you lug with you will make your trip less fun, and fun is the whole point of your endeavor.

> **Anything extra you lug with you will make your trip less fun, and fun is the whole point of your endeavor.**

The basic idea of ultralight backpacking with kids is to pare your load to its essentials, then look to each of those essentials for ways to lighten them. Gear-wise, you'll get the most out of what you spend by investing in lightweight packs, sleeping bags, pads, tent, and food. The next level will involve investing in lightweight clothing, boots, and cookware.

Bring only the clothes you and your kids wear, extra layers for warmth and rain, sleeping gear and shelter, kitchen supplies, and the bare minimum of toiletries, first-aid items, and essentials such as bug repellent and sunscreen.

Bring nothing else.

Don't carry extra clothes. Kid backpacking trips are, by necessity, relatively short affairs. Be willing to get a little smelly during your trip. Your shoulders and back will thank you for it.

Don't bring time-passers such as books and pocket-size games. Instead, spend your free time actively playing with your kids—something there's never time enough for at home.

As noted later in this chapter, running water makes a terrific toy. When there's no water around, Sue and I often play a rock-toss game with Taylor and Logan that the four of us have developed together. The game is nothing more than a wilderness version of bowling. We stack five or six flat, hockey-puck-size rocks on top of one another, then choose fist-size "shooter" rocks to toss at the stack. Distances from which shots are taken are handicapped

What You'll Have to Carry and Who Will Do the Carrying

For three-day, two-night backpacking trips, Sue and I and our boys carry roughly 80 pounds between us, with the boys gradually carrying more of that total each year as they grow bigger and stronger, and Sue and I carrying commensurably less as we grow older and more decrepit. That 80 pounds roughly breaks down like this:

■ 10 pounds: combined weight of four ultralight packs.

■ 20 pounds: lightweight tent or tents, sleeping bags, and pads.

■ 12 pounds: coats, rainwear, and extra clothing layers.

■ 8 pounds: kitchen, toiletry, and miscellaneous supplies.

■ 30 pounds: food, fuel, and two to three liters of water for hiking between water sources.

Using Taylor, Logan, and other children with whom Sue and I have backpacked as guides, here are some very rough amounts you can count on your kids carrying:

■ At age 5 or 6, up to 10 pounds each for a mile or two, at which point their little packs will become uncomfortable and you'll end up strapping them atop yours.

■ By age 8, they'll carry the same 10 pounds or a little more for several miles without complaint.

■ At age 10, they'll proudly carry up to 20 pounds.

■ At age 12, they'll be ready for 25 or even 30 pounds.

based on age and ability level to make each game as even as possible.

Players take turns "shooting," or tossing, their shooters at the pile of flat rocks. Players score 10 points for each flat rock they knock from the stack with their shooters, up to a full 50 or 60 points if they knock over the entire stack. The first player to reach a predetermined point total wins.

Our rock-toss game is nothing special. It's merely one of many such possibilities that will enable you to pleasantly pass time with your kids in camp during a backpacking trip.

Go Short

There's no need to go great distances into the backcountry for your kids to feel as if they're in the middle of nowhere.

When Logan was a toddler and Taylor not much older, the longest family backpacking trip Sue and I could manage was

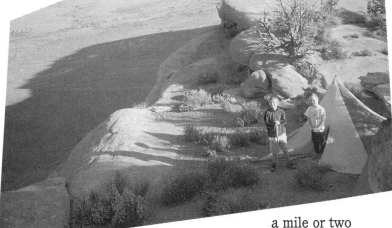

a mile or two from the trailhead. Such trips were plenty for the boys. Besides, as far as they were concerned, the moment they were out of sight of the car, they were as deep in the wilderness as if they had traveled 20 miles from the nearest road.

Not until Logan reached age 5 did we begin taking family backpacking trips of any significant length. At that age, we learned, kids are capable of fairly long trips into the backcountry. As a kindergartner, for example, Logan completed a number of multiday backpacking trips. Logan's kindergarten-year trips involved hiking up to 7 miles on a given day and carrying about 10 pounds of water and gear in his little-kid daypack.

(Note that as your kids grow older, they'll quickly be capable of some pretty serious miles and vertical feet with packs on their backs. On a recent Grand Canyon backpacking trip, Logan at age 8 hiked 8 miles and 4200 vertical feet out of the canyon on the final day of the trip, without complaint or hardship.)

MAKE TWO TRIPS

If your trip is short enough, you can return to the car to bring in a second load. Such a process may be the only way for you to get away from your car for a night when your kids are babies and toddlers.

Hike-in campsites are common in California state parks and Canadian national and provincial parks, and are found in many other federal, state, and county parks in the US. Such campsites, generally less than a mile from the parking lot, provide a perfect opportunity for you to take your very young children backpacking.

Hike-in campsites provide perfect opportunities for you to take your very young children backpacking.

CAMP AT WATER SOURCES

Sue and I have done a few desert backpacking trips with Taylor and Logan to dry campsites. Though the trips were perfectly enjoyable, they weren't as fun for the boys or for us as camping near water.

Lakes, creeks, and rivers provide endless play opportunities for you and your kids. Take full advantage of them. Don't be tempted to camp away from water on a bluff or ridge for the view. Kids don't care much about views. They want to play.

Dry campsites are especially daunting because they require ranging quite a ways to find water after you arrive in camp, or carrying all the water you'll need with you, which means you and your kids will have to carry heavy loads and will be limited to an overnighter.

Possibilities

HIKE-IN CAMPSITES

Hike-in campsites provide great opportunities for you and your kids to try backpacking for the first time.

Though located up a trail and away from roads, hike-in sites generally include such amenities as picnic tables, critter-control food boxes, and bathrooms. In many parks, hike-in campsites never fill up. Conversely, sites in some parks are extremely popular.

A few years ago, Sue and I applied for and received a permit months in advance to camp with our boys in one of the five highly sought-after hike-in campsites on the half of Maine's remote Isle au Haut that is part of Acadia National Park (www.nps.gov/acad). We loaded our packs, caught a mail boat to the island, and hiked to our site, which included a covered shelter for our tent. Our night on the undeveloped, uninhabited half of the island far from roads and cars was terrific for the entirely different backwoods world it presented us. My family is accustomed to the dry Southwest backcountry. As such, the experience was well worth the months of advance planning and scheduling it required.

In addition to Isle au Haut, other popular ferry-in/hike-in campsites include those on Angel Island in San Francisco Bay (www.angelisland.org) and on Orcas Island, one of the San Juan Islands in Washington's Puget Sound (www.orcasisland.org).

Among hundreds of popular drive-to-the-trailhead/hike-in campsites are those amid the towering redwoods of the Little River Valley in Van Damme State Park near Mendocino on the northern California coast (www.parks.ca.gov; keywords: Van Damme), and in the rugged western half of the Shawnee National Forest in southern Illinois at Johnson Creek Recreation Area (www.fs.fed.us; keyword: Shawnee).

It's easy to use an internet search engine to locate hike-in campsites near your home or along the route of a planned vacation. Listings for hike-in sites in Iowa, Wisconsin, Minnesota, Illinois, Hawaii, Michigan,

California, Washington, Texas, North Carolina, Missouri, and Arkansas were among the first few dozen of the more than 15,000 hits that resulted from a search I conducted for "hike-in campsites."

POPULAR- AND SHORT-TRAIL TRIPS

The next step up from hike-in campsites is short backpack trips and/or trips on popular trails to undeveloped campsites, either reserved sites or those of your choosing. Finding popular trails to backpack with your kids is easy, but getting permits for them often requires advance planning.

Before we hiked the Grand Canyon (www.nps.gov/grca) with Taylor and Logan, Sue and I got started backpacking with them by regularly reserving and backpacking to preassigned backcountry sites—none more than a couple of miles from the trailhead—in the Needles District of Canyonlands National Park in southeastern Utah (www.nps.gov/cany).

Other popular and less demanding backpacking trails that are great for kids include:

Pinkham Notch to Tuckerman Ravine: On the east side of Mt. Washington in New Hampshire (www.tuckerman.org).

Appalachian Trail: Virtually any stretch from Georgia to Maine (www.appalachiantrail.org).

National Parks: Well-trodden trails in any number of popular national parks such as Yosemite in California, Glacier in Montana, Yellowstone in Wyoming, and Shenandoah in Virginia (www.nps.gov).

Pacific Crest Trail: Spur trails leading to the most popular sections of the Pacific Crest Trail and overlapping John Muir Trail along the spine of California's southern Sierra (www.pcta.org).

QUIET-TRAIL TRIPS

Suitable quiet trails for backpacking with your kids are peculiar to particular users. Are you and/or your kids birders? Peak baggers? History buffs? These and other specifics such as the ages and hiking abilities of your children will determine the types of less-traveled trails you'll want to seek out.

To further narrow things down, consult maps, employees of local outdoor stores, and local, small-print-run guidebooks. Also, try internet searches using the name of the state or region that interests you coupled with the word "trails."

If you find potential trails close to home, consider driving there to check them out during trail runs or dayhikes to see if they offer what you want before taking your kids backpacking on them.

MULTIDAY TRIPS

Opportunities for you to take multiday backpacking trips with your kids as they grow older probably will be limited.

You'll likely be able to squeeze in only one lengthy backpacking trip with your kids each year. If you figure you won't be able to do such ambitious trips with your kids until they reach age 10 or 12, that means you'll have the opportunity for only half a dozen or so annual, multiday backpacking trips with them before they're grown and gone.

Given that reality, you may want to focus on some of the best-known backpacking trips in the country when you consider which lengthy trips to tackle with your kids. Some of the biggest of the big-time backpacking trips in the US include:

Long Trail: A section of Vermont's 270-mile Long Trail (www.greenmountainclub.org), the oldest long-distance hiking trail in America.

John Muir Trail: A section of the 211-mile John Muir Trail (www.pcta.org), which runs between Yosemite Valley and Mt. Whitney in California, encompassing what many consider the finest mountain scenery in the US.

Cirque of the Towers: The renowned hike into this remote region (www.visitsublettecounty.com) in Wyoming's Wind River Mountains. (Be prepared for thick mosquitoes in July and August, and early- and late-season storms and snow in June and September.)

Colorado Trail or Continental Divide Trail: Any of the rugged and beautiful southern sections of the 487-mile Colorado Trail (www.coloradotrail.org), or a portion of the Continental Divide Trail (www.cdtrail.org) in the remote Weminuche Wilderness Area of the San Juan Mountains, both in southwestern Colorado.

Grand Canyon: Any number of trail options (www.nps.gov/grca).

Grand Gulch Primitive Area: A trip to explore the many ancient Indian ruins of southeastern Utah's Grand Gulch (www.ut.blm.gov/monticello).

Wonderland Trail: A portion of the 93-mile hike around Washington's Mt. Rainier (www.nps.gov/mora).

Denali National Park: A multiday, trail-free adventure on the tundra among the grizzlies in Alaska (www.nps.gov/dena).

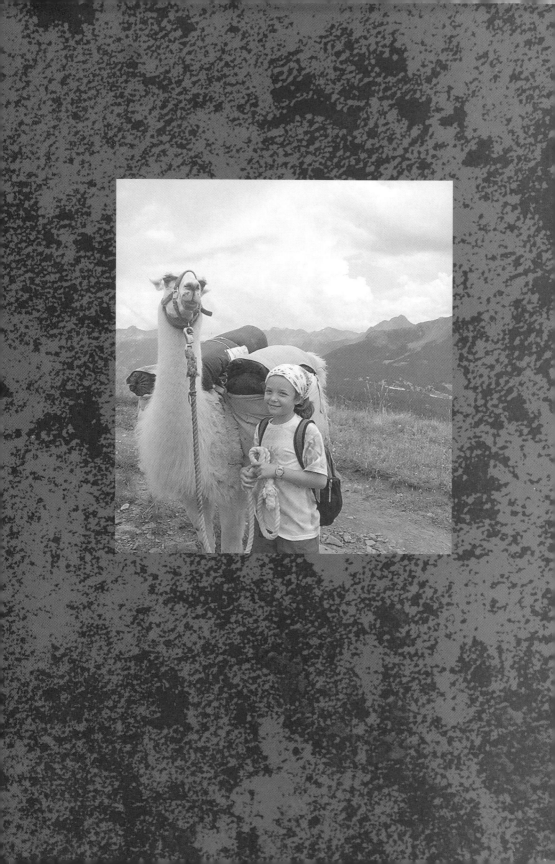

Backpacking Made Easier:
15 Llama Trekking and Hut Trips

When it comes to journeying into the backcountry on foot, Sue and I have stuck with the simplicity of backpacking with our boys—so far. The older we get, however, the more our backs and knees are paying the price of our decision.

Tired of paying that price and interested in trying something new, several families we know have taken llama treks into the backcountry using rental llamas, with uniformly great results.

The other way to make backpacking easier (not to mention more comfortable) is to take advantage of the many backcountry cabins and yurts—those round, canvas structures—around the country.

Llama Treks

Llama-supported treks, whether self-run or outfitter-run, combine the gear-hauling capability of river trips with the freedom to go where you want in the backcountry.

Llamas can carry up to 100 pounds of gear each, enabling you to throw in virtually all the treats you ever dreamed of carrying on a backpacking trip but nixed as too heavy. All that extra kid stuff? Sure. Extra-large family tent? Absolutely. Ham and eggs for breakfast? No problem.

"Llama trekking pretty much appeals to everybody," says Stuart Wilde, owner of Wild Earth Llama Adventures in Taos, New Mexico. "You get to explore the beauty and wonder of the wilderness without carrying a heavy pack. What could be better?"

Moreover, Wilde points out, "Llamas are the perfect high-altitude, low-impact animal. They exemplify the low-impact, leave-no-trace ethic of backcountry travel."

Unlike horses' hooves, llamas' padded feet are easy on trails—easier, even, than human foot traffic. No food must be carried into the backcountry for llamas; they eat vegetation along the way.

Lucy Lowe, owner of English Mountain Llama Treks in Hot Springs, North Carolina, says, "Llamas' surefootedness, common sense, and gentle manner make them excellent pack animals and trail companions."

Llamas have been domesticated for more than 6000 years. They're great with children. Kids can, and normally do, lead their own assigned llamas along a trail on backcountry trips. That's a way cool thing for kids to do. Plus, when kids are leading their llamas along a trail, they tend to forget about the fact that they're actually trudging along the same trail themselves.

"Llamas create a diversion and a responsibility so kids are occupied," says Wilde. "They don't notice being tired and they're not bored."

DO-IT-YOURSELF LLAMA TREKKING

More and more do-it-yourself types are taking rental llamas into the backcountry these days. The animals are welcome wherever horses are allowed, including wilderness areas.

"I can't imagine a better kid trip," says Eric Pierson, who took a rental-llama trip with his wife, Cathy, and children, Carly, then 8, and Chase, then 6. The Pierson family joined another family to hike a portion of the Colorado Trail in south-central Colorado with a pair of rental llamas for gear-hauling support.

Each llama cost $40 per day to rent. The Piersons transported the two animals to and from the trailhead in their own trailer. Having the llamas' owner provide that service would have added $100 to the total cost.

Before they left the llama ranch with the animals, the owner showed the two families how to load and picket the animals. Then it was off to the trailhead.

"They were a dream on the trail," Eric says. "They were never forceful. They just cruised right along with us. We never felt like we had to urge them up steep parts of the trail or worry about them running us over when we went downhill."

Carly and Chase loved leading the animals. "In fact, we couldn't even get any time on the leads," Pierson says. "The kids wanted to keep hold of them the whole time."

The Basics

- Llama trekking and hut trips make it easier to get into the backcountry with your kids than back-packing.

- Do-it-yourself and guided llama trips are available in more and more locations across the country.

- Backcountry cabins and yurts are increasingly available for hike-in trips as well.

Each day, Eric reports, the kids uncomplainingly put in double the hiking miles they would have willingly hiked during a normal backpacking trip.

As for the adults? "All we had to carry were light day-packs, and we just did that for convenience," Eric says. "The llamas carried everything else."

A huge thunderstorm swept toward them one afternoon of the trip. In camp, the first-time llama trekkers eyed the approaching thunderstorm with concern, wondering how the llamas would react.

They needn't have worried. "The storm hit with lots of lightning and huge thunder," Eric remembers, "but the lla-mas just sat in the grass and never responded to it at all."

In a word, says Pierson, his family's do-it-yourself llama trek was "terrific."

Because self-supported llama trekking is relatively new, rental llamas aren't yet widely available. You'll have to work the internet and phone to learn whether rental lla-mas are available in the area you want to visit.

Llama owners rent their animals only to experienced backcountry travelers. Rental rates range from $40 to $50 per day, plus drop-off and pick-up fees based on mileage.

163

Outfitter-supported llama trekking is fairly common. No matter where in the country you wish to explore the backcountry, you'll likely find a llama outfitter willing to take you there.

To learn more about llamas in general, visit www.llama.org. Though the site is aimed at llama owners and those who aspire to own llamas, it provides much good information for potential llama renters, including the story of a Pennsylvania couple who llama-trekked for two months with their two young children along 500 miles of the Continental Divide Trail in Montana.

Hut Trips

Backcountry huts are widely available in many national forests, with more being added as demand increases. Hut trips offer families a different set of benefits than llama trekking. Unlike llama trips, you and your kids will be responsible for carrying on your own back everything you need for a hut trip. But, unlike backpacking, you won't have to carry tents, cookware, and, in some cases, food. As a result, your packs will be lighter than those you must carry on a fully self-supported backpacking trip. That means you'll be able to hike farther into the backcountry or explore more along the way.

The trade-off of a hut trip, of course, is that you'll be staying in an established structure on a heavily used site as opposed to tent camping in a less-used location. Still, most yurts and many smaller cabins can be rented in their entirety, making them and their backcountry sites the sole province of your hiking party. Moreover, rather than undertaking a potentially arduous multiday hut-to-hut trip with kids, you can rent a single hut and use it as a base from which to take dayhikes, climbs, and fishing excursions. And you can share a hut with one or more other families, turning your backcountry trip into a kid-filled free-for-all. Such trips offer the high fun quotient of multi-family rafting trips without all the gear demands and required water-travel knowledge of self-supported river journeys.

Unlike do-it-yourself llama treks, do-it-yourself hut trips are the rule as opposed to the exception. There are a few guided backcountry hut-to-hut trips out there, but hut trips, for the most part, are on-your-own affairs. Taking a hut trip is a simple matter of deciding what region of the country you want to explore, then working the internet and guidebooks to find huts, whether in the form of cabins or yurts.

You'll want to look for huts that aren't too deep in the backcountry or too many vertical feet above a given trailhead. Three miles in on a trail involving no more than 1500 vertical feet of elevation gain is probably all you'll want to tackle with children under 10. If your kids are in the 10- to 12-year-old range, you can bump those numbers up some. If your kids are in their teen years, you'll need to consider *your* endurance limits rather than theirs when it comes to deciding how far into the backcountry you want to hike.

Possibilities

ENGLISH MOUNTAIN LLAMA TREKS

Lucy Lowe and Laura Higgins, co-owners of the Hot Springs, North Carolina-based English Mountain Llama Treks, offer one of the best family backcountry adventures in the South: a llama-supported trip into Panthertown Valley in far western North Carolina's Nantahala National Forest.

Panthertown is a broad valley in the Smoky Mountains famous for its 200- to 300-foot granite domes. Views from the uplifted domes are tremendous. The sides of the domes make for great rock climbing, which explains why the valley is known as the Yosemite of the East. The three creeks that flow through Panthertown Valley are studded with kid-friendly swimming holes and slide rocks.

All children on English Mountain's Panthertown trips are assigned their own llamas to lead. Food and all camping supplies are provided on the trips, which can be either one or two nights in length.

Lowe says the outfitter's Panthertown trip is popular with single parents who want to give their children a taste of the backcountry but can't pull off a family backpacking trip on their own. In many cases, Lowe says, English Mountain teams include more than one single- or double-parent family on Panthertown trips. Lowe says doing so enriches the experience for everyone involved.

"The kids—may of whom never have slept in the outdoors before—work and play together and come off the trips as best friends," Lowe says.

Children as young as 6 are welcome on English Mountain's llama treks, which range in cost from $230 to $350. For more information, contact English Mountain at 828-622-9686 or go to www.hikinginthesmokies.com.

WILD EARTH LLAMA ADVENTURES

When Stuart Wilde's oldest child, now a teenager, was a baby, Wilde bought a pair of llamas on a payment plan so he could continue to visit the backcountry areas he loved in northern New Mexico with his baby and all the gear the baby required. Wilde enjoyed it so much, he went on to found Wild Earth Llama Adventures in Taos, New Mexico. In the years since, Wilde and his wife, Leah, have taken more than a thousand trekkers on llama-supported trips into the northern New Mexico wilderness.

Because of their experience trekking with babies in the backcountry, the Wildes welcome infants. All of Wild Earth's offerings are family oriented and custom designed to best fit the ages and abilities of the children and adult family members involved.

"A normal Wild Earth trip involves a leisurely hike to a base camp at about 11,000 feet," Wilde says. "Then we do dayhikes and climbs on subsequent days. I break out a map and present options based on what I think is appropriate. I'll suggest easier hikes for families with kids who are 5 or 6, and more strenuous hikes for families with older kids. We tend to save the most strenuous hikes and peak climbs as a way to cap the ends of our trips."

Wilde says he works hard to make sure the trips are fun for children.

"When they're adults," says Wilde, "I want the kids we take along to say, 'I went hiking and camping with my family when I was a kid. I loved it and I'm still doing it.'"

Wild Earth trips run between two and six days in length and begin at $250. For more information about Wild Earth, call 800-758-5262 or visit www.llamaadventures.com.

APPALACHIAN TRAIL HUTS

According to Appalachian Mountain Club (AMC) public affairs director Rob Burbank, the AMC's eight dormitory-style cabins strung along the Appalachian Trail high in the White Mountains of New Hampshire are "an unparalleled system of huts, available to young and old, in some of the nation's most breathtaking locations." As such, the huts offer a perfect way to introduce your kids to foot travel in the backcountry.

Dinner, breakfast, blankets, and pillows are provided at the huts. You and your kids need only hike from cabin to cabin (or simply into one cabin and back out again) with

167

clothing, lightweight sleep sacks, and lunch food on your backs.

Educational programs, many just for kids, are offered by the hut employees each evening. In addition to those programs, your children will meet thru-hikers on the Appalachian Trail as well as other backpackers kicking up their heels in the woods, which will get your kids enthused about backcountry hiking and backpacking. A single trip along any portion of the AMC's hut system may well be all it takes to get you and your kids psyched to try a full-on backpacking trip in the wilderness. An AMC hut trip will also serve as a terrific, away-from-the-car family adventure in its own right.

Like the AMC huts, Colorado's 10th Mountain Division huts are great for families introducing their kids to backpacking.

The AMC's historic eight-hut system, more than a century old, stretches along the most scenic portion of the Appalachian Trail. The huts are open from June to October. (June is black-fly season.)

The easiest hut to reach is less than 3 miles from the nearest trailhead via a gentle trail. Families are welcome to use huts as base camps; in fact, rates are discounted for stays of three nights or longer.

Note that the huts are big. They sleep up to 90 people and can be noisy.

Shuttles to and from various trailheads are available. Cost of the huts, with meals, is about $80 per night for adults and $50 for kids. Reservations are required. For more information, call 603-466-2727 or go to www.outdoors.org/lodging/huts.

10TH MOUNTAIN DIVISION HUTS

The premier hut system in the country is run by the 10th Mountain Division Hut Association in the heart of the central Colorado Rockies. The association manages 29 huts connected by 350 miles of trails in four national forests. The hut system is named in honor of the 10th Mountain Division of the US Army, members of which trained at Camp Hale in central Colorado.

Many of the huts can be reached by kids. The primary challenge for many 10th Mountain hut-to-hut hikers is altitude. Hut locations range in elevation from 10,000 to

12,000 feet. If you live at or near sea level, be sure to spend some time with your kids acclimatizing in the mountains before beginning your hut trip.

Like the trips to the Appalachian Mountain Club's huts, visiting 10th Mountain Division huts provides a great opportunity to introduce your children to the idea of backpacking. However, a 10th Mountain hut trip will require more of you and your kids than an AMC hut trip. Unlike the AMC huts, meals and blankets are not supplied at 10th Mountain huts, so you'll need to carry food and sleeping bags with you. Utensils, wood stoves for heating, propane stoves for cooking, and photovoltaic power for lighting are provided.

Most 10th Mountain huts accommodate about 16 people in a common area and shared rooms that sleep three or four. Cost is roughly $30 per night for adults; children 12 and younger stay for half price.

One of the easiest huts to reach is the Shrine Mountain Inn, actually a group of three huts (with a shared sauna) less than 3 hiking miles from Interstate 70 at the top of Vail Pass west of Denver. A trip with your kids to Shrine Mountain Inn or any number of other 10th Mountain huts would make a fine adventurous addition to a Rocky Mountain family vacation.

More than 10,000 people stay in the 10th Mountain huts each summer season, which begins on or about July 1 and runs through September 30. Reservations made far in advance are essential. For more information, call 970-925-5775 or go to www.huts.org.

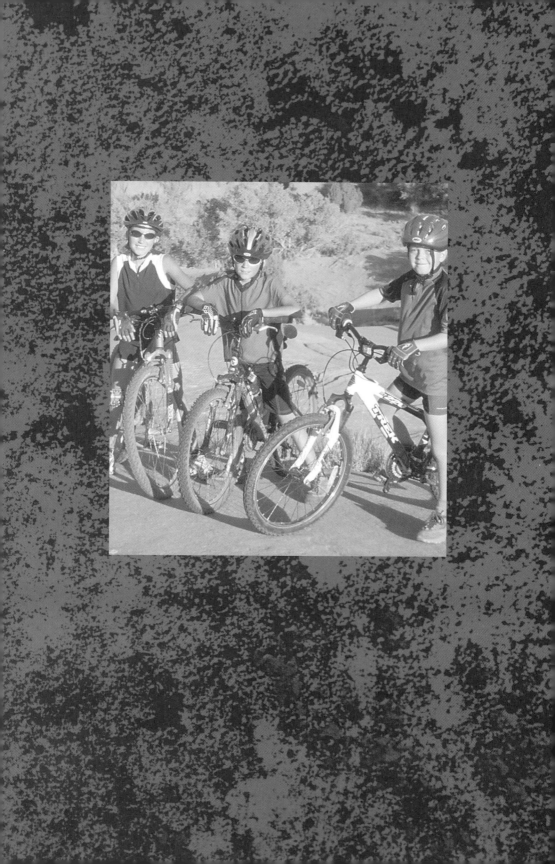

16 Mountain Biking

A dad I know was so gaga for mountain biking that he couldn't sit still when his first baby reached toddler age. He stuck a helmet on her head, belted her into a car seat, and bungeed the car seat into a pull-behind bike trailer. He then set out to learn just how much "single track," or trail, mountain biking he could do while pulling a two-wheeled bike trailer behind him.

The answer, it turns out, is quite a bit—especially if you're built like a New York Giants linebacker, which this guy is, and have thighs that approximate those of Lance Armstrong, which this guy does. My friend rode trails so gnarly that the trailer carrying his daughter regularly flipped sideways on tight turns. Once, in fact, the trailer broke free of my friend's bike and did an entire roll.

"Thing is, she loved it," my friend said of his daughter. "She screamed with delight every time the trailer flipped on its side, and she really loved it when she did that roll."

I've never been one for turning my kids into real-life bobble-head dolls. Still, my friend's story illustrates the lengths to which some parents will go to keep pursuing the outdoor sports they love A.C. (After Children), and the pleasure kids take, even as nonparticipants, in those sports.

The great thing about mountain biking with your kids is that, like dayhiking, you can do it just about anywhere there's a dirt road or suitable trail. Though mountain biking requires more gear than dayhiking, it doesn't involve the high degree of skills and more limited locations required by outdoor sports such as rock climbing, whitewater kayaking, and river running.

The Basics

- The progression from pulling your toddler behind you in a trailer to watching your pre-teen leave you in the dust is a quick one when it comes to mountain biking.

- Your kids will be capable of true mountain biking on trails and slickrock when they're as young as 6.

- There's good reason Moab, Utah, constitutes hallowed ground when it comes to mountain biking, but many other regions of the country are terrific for family mountain biking adventures as well.

- If you're new to biking and/or to outdoor adventuring, guided mountain biking trips offer terrific and fun ways for you to get out into the backcountry with your kids.

Once you and your kids are appropriately outfitted (see "Gear Talk," page 174), you can throw your bikes on your car rack and head out for a day ride on little more than a moment's notice. Conversely, you and your kids can make an entire vacation out of mountain biking. If you're a do-it-yourselfer, you can drive to one of the meccas of mountain biking—Moab, Utah, perhaps, or Crested Butte, Colorado—and spend the bulk of your vacation riding with your kids. You can also fly to one of the meccas and rent gear for the extent of your vacation, much like renting ski gear for a ski vacation. Or you can sign up with an outfitter for an organized trip that includes gear.

Getting Rolling

Like our friend with the bobble-head daughter, Sue and I were dedicated mountain bikers long before Taylor and Logan came along. We missed mountain biking while our boys were little and got them started in the sport as quickly as we could.

At age 5, Taylor began riding the miniature six-speed mountain bike we picked up for him. At first he used it to tag along with us on dirt roads and level trails near our home. Not long after he turned 6, he graduated to riding his tiny bike on short portions of the Slickrock Trail in

Moab. After that, there was no stopping him—nor Logan, who followed Taylor's pedal strokes two years later.

One recent family trip Sue and I took with Taylor and Logan is worth noting as you consider the mountain biking trips you might wish to do with your kids. Our trip was a multiday backcountry tour following the route of one of Western Spirit Cycling Adventures' family mountain

The Best Rides, By Age

When you want to get your kids started mountain biking, keep in mind the following guidelines to determine whether a certain trip is appropriate for the age of your child:

■ Dirt-road (or "double track") riding is great when your kids are toddlers and can ride in pull-behind trailers (no added car seats and bungee cords required).

■ You can go on double-track and level single-track rides with your preschool-age kids on attached trail-a-bikes, especially those with gears and shock absorbers. "I definitely had to move up to a trail-a-bike with a shock," a friend told me. "[My daughter] kept bouncing off the first one I got."

■ Off-pavement double-track and level single-track riding is fine to do with your 5- to 7-year-old kids.

■ Moderate to advanced single-track riding is appropriate with your 8- or 9-year-olds as they gain more control over their bikes.

■ By the time your kids are 10 or 11, you will be trying desperately to keep up on stretches of steep, rocky single track as they blast up the trail, leaving you flailing behind.

■ Finally, you'll cringe in terror as you watch your kids, in their early teens, try their first freeriding moves.

biking adventures—this one just across the state line from our Colorado home in southeastern Utah.

Rather than go with Western Spirit on what the company calls its Trail of the Ancients adventure, we self-supported the trip. The boys rode the entire route while Sue and I traded off riding with them and driving our pickup as a sag wagon. Over the course of four days, the boys

Gear Talk

Good mountain bikes are a major financial investment. A basic full-suspension bike runs $1000, and that's before you throw in clipless pedals and shoes. Add a helmet, biking clothes, and a Camelbak, and you'll easily approach $1500. And that's just for you, never mind your kids.

If you're new to mountain biking, the best way to start is by renting. If you do decide to gear up, you'll save significant money by buying quality used gear or shopping for new gear at end-of-season sales.

Here are some other suggestions:

1. Don't buy bikes that are too big for your kids. You'll only end up with frustrated children riding bikes that are not safe for them. Better to buy high-quality used bikes and resell them when your kids outgrow them.

   If you get your kids started mountain biking early, you'll be looking at three preadolescent bike purchases as they grow:

   - Ages 5 to 8: A small, six- or seven-speed bike with 20-inch wheels. Price: about $200.

   - Ages 9 to 11: A midsize bike with 24-inch wheels and 18 to 21 speeds. Price: about $300.

   - Early teens: A small-framed adult bike with 26-inch wheels. Price: $500 and up.

2. If your kids get serious about mountain biking, don't be afraid to get them clipless pedals as soon as they move up to a 26-inch bike. Those pedals will make increasingly difficult trails easier.

3. Invest in good helmets with sun visors.

4. Insist that your kids wear sunglasses when riding single-track trails to avoid injuries caused by branches that might otherwise poke them in the eye.

5. Good hydration is as important to kid mountain bikers as it is to adults. Camelbaks or Camelbak knockoffs make great presents.

6. Pick up stylin' jerseys and bike shorts for your kid riders. They'll love looking the part of a "real" mountain biker, and they may be more likely to stick with the sport as a result.

rode 70 miles of rough, remote four-wheel-drive roads through stunning country. The roads were carefully picked by the experts at Western Spirit for their mountain and desert scenery, lack of motorized vehicle use, and suitability for mountain biking.

If you're a do-it-yourself type, following the route of one of Western Spirit's trips may be as good an option for you as it was for us. Of course, simply joining one of Western Spirit's family trips is a great way to go as well.

Another good starter option is to rent bikes for a day at a ski area. You can then ride the lift to the top of the mountain with your kids and rented bikes, and take off from there. Virtually all ski areas rent mountain bikes during the summer months. It's worth noting, however, that mountain bike rentals are generally available only down to the smallest adult-size frame with 26-inch wheels, which are appropriate for good-sized 10-year-olds and up. For anything smaller—a bike with 24-inch or 20-inch wheels—you'll be faced with providing your own.

You can also contact mountain biking clubs and organizations in your area such as the New England Mountain

Bike Association (www.nemba.org) and its many local chapters for suggestions, local tips, and dates of group "fun" rides. The International Mountain Bicycling Association sponsors an annual Take a Kid Mountain Biking Day. The event, held at sites around the country on the first Saturday in October, provides an excellent opportunity to introduce mountain biking to your kids in the company of other youngsters. See www.imba.com for the site nearest you.

Freeriding

If you spend much time mountain biking with your kids, the subject of freeriding—extreme mountain biking—is sure to come up.

In recent years, mostly male teens and 20-somethings have been tricking out their mountain bikes with heavy-duty components, then using their beefed-up bikes to jump off cliffs (called "wheelie drops"), ride log bridges, and conquer formerly unrideable sections of back-country, both on-trail and, to the consternation of many, off.

Having seen the potential for profit

offered by the new sport, mountain bike manufacturers
have developed freeride-specific mountain bikes and
released them to the masses.

With youngsters and bikes, just about anything counts
as freeriding. Descending steep inclines, jumping small
logs, splashing through puddles—any bit of mountain biking can be "freeriding" for your kids if you declare it so.

Using the term to encourage your kids to challenge
themselves on their mountain bikes may not be a bad
idea. Just be prepared for the day they ask you to buy
them freeride bikes so they can really go freeriding. If you
and your kids are curious to learn more about freeriding,
visit www.mtb-freeride.com.

> **Any bit of mountain biking can be "freeriding" for your youngsters if you declare it so.**

Possibilities

MOAB

Nothing beats mountain biking the official Slickrock
Trail and other incredible slickrock routes around Moab,
Utah. Yes, Moab is overrun with mountain bikers (and
Jeepers and ATVers for that matter), but for good reason.

Sue and I have biked Moab's smooth sandstone trails
regularly since the mid-'80s. Crowded as the slickrock
around Moab has become, we still head there with Taylor
and Logan as often as we can. Riding Moab's slickrock is
too fun to let the crowds scare us away.

If you really want to get your kids jazzed about mountain biking, take them on a mountain biking vacation to
Moab, which is the center of the mountain biking uni-
verse. One particular multiday mountain biking trip in the
Moab area is worth considering: The 100-mile White Rim
Road, often called the White Rim Trail, follows four-
wheel-drive roads through a remote section of
Canyonlands National Park on rock shelves above the
Green and Colorado rivers. Families and groups of families
often ride and camp along the route in do-it-yourself fashion by providing their own sag wagons, which parents
take turns driving, and in which youngsters—tired of riding—spend time as passengers.

The five members of the Lloyd family, including father-son canyoneers Leo and Kendall (see page 136), have ridden the White Rim annually since Kendall was a 7-year-old who spent most of his first "ride" in the sag wagon. Kendall now has ridden the White Rim six times. The last time he rode it, at age 13, he pedaled the entire route.

Private-party permits to ride the White Rim must be secured via lottery as much as a year in advance. For details, go to www.nps.gov/cany (keywords: Explore the Park). Outfitters such as Moab's Rim Tours (www.rim-tours.com) also run trips on the White Rim. Visit www.discovermoab.com for more information about the region.

Many locales other than Moab and Crested Butte offer great mountain biking and are worth a visit with kids.

CRESTED BUTTE

Was mountain biking founded in Crested Butte, Colorado, or in Marin County, California? The debate still rages. Crested Butte, however, offers plenty of charms for a family mountain biking vacation.

Located at the head of the Gunnison River valley in the heart of the central Colorado Rockies, tiny Crested Butte offers oodles of serpentine summertime single-track rides heading into the backcountry in all directions from its four-block-long, Disneyland-perfect Victorian downtown.

If the riding alone isn't enough, try visiting the Mountain Bike Hall of Fame in town to further stoke your kids' enthusiasm for the sport. For more information about Crested Butte and the Mountain Bike Hall of Fame, visit www.visitcrestedbutte.com and www.mtnbikehalloffame.com.

OTHER MECCAS-ON-THE-MAKE

Arguably, Moab offers the finest mountain biking, and Crested Butte the finest "mountain" mountain biking, on the planet. But other locales around the country offer great mountain biking as well, and many of these places are worth a visit with kids. Two websites, www.mbronline.com (keyword: Destinations), and www.gorp.away.com (keywords: Beyond Moab), offer tantalizing looks at a few of these meccas-on-the-make.

The best of the up-and-comers in the East is West Virginia (www.bicyclewv.com). *Mountain Biking* magazine rates West Virginia as one of the top five mountain biking destinations in the country. The compact mountainous state is known for its challenging—and, admittedly, wet—rides on single track and logging roads.

The two best riding locations in West Virginia are the protected, 70,000-acre New River Gorge (www.nps.gov/neri), and the 900,000-acre Monongahela National Forest (www.fs.fed.us; keyword: Monongahela).

Other meccas-on-the-make include Bend, Oregon (www.visitbend.com); Sun Valley, Idaho (www.visitsunvalley.com); Custer, South Dakota (www.custersd.com), Park City, Utah (www.parkcityinfo.com); and my hometown, Durango, Colorado (www.durango.org).

WESTERN SPIRIT CYCLING ADVENTURES' FAMILY MOUNTAIN BIKING TRIPS

There's probably no better way to experience backcountry mountain biking with your children than on one of Moab, Utah-based Western Spirit's five-day, four-night family trips. The easygoing trips are pure fun for kids and adults alike.

The trips run $700 to $900 per person. Those prices include all food, gear, and transportation to and from a town near each trip's start and end points. Child care is included for parents who want to get in some extra riding while their kids hang out in camp. Children as young as 2 are welcome on the trips, which are tailored to meet the needs and wants of participants.

Western Spirit currently offers eight family-specific backcountry mountain biking trips each summer, with more in the offing. The eight trips are scattered across the country, many near mountain biking hot spots discussed earlier in this chapter. The company offers two trips in Wyoming's Yellowstone/Grand Teton region, two in Utah's canyon country, and one trip each in California's redwoods, West Virginia's mountains, South Dakota's Black Hills, and Arizona's Grand Canyon area.

Every Western Spirit family trip features day rides spiced with non-biking activities such as a hike to an ancient Indian ruin or a ride on a steam-powered train. Evenings are busy with skits, coyote-howling contests, and other campfire-based activities.

Western Spirit offered its first family trip in 2000. The Moab-based outfitter's eight trips now account for a third of the company's business. Why have Western Spirit's family trips taken off? Certainly the outfitter is riding the same wave of interest in family vacations as the rest of the travel industry.

But Western Spirit's added secret, owner Ashley Korenblat believes, is its emphasis on the "extreme" aspects of biking trips. The kids on Western Spirit's trips don't leap off 20-foot cliffs on freeride bikes. Rather, the company finds the word "extreme" in a less outrageous way—in simply making each of its family trips as back-country-oriented as possible. Unlike adult mountain biking trips offered by other outfitters that feature day rides followed by cushy nights in inns and bed-and-breakfasts, Western Spirit's family mountain biking trips are all about experiencing the outdoors. Not only do the trips involve camping; as often as possible, they involve camping at backcountry sites far from campgrounds, pavement, and crowds.

Western Spirit's family trips sell out quickly each year. If you want to go on one of the trips with your kids, you'll have to plan ahead and ante up your deposit money early. For more information about Western Spirit, call 800-845-2453 or go to www.westernspirit.com.

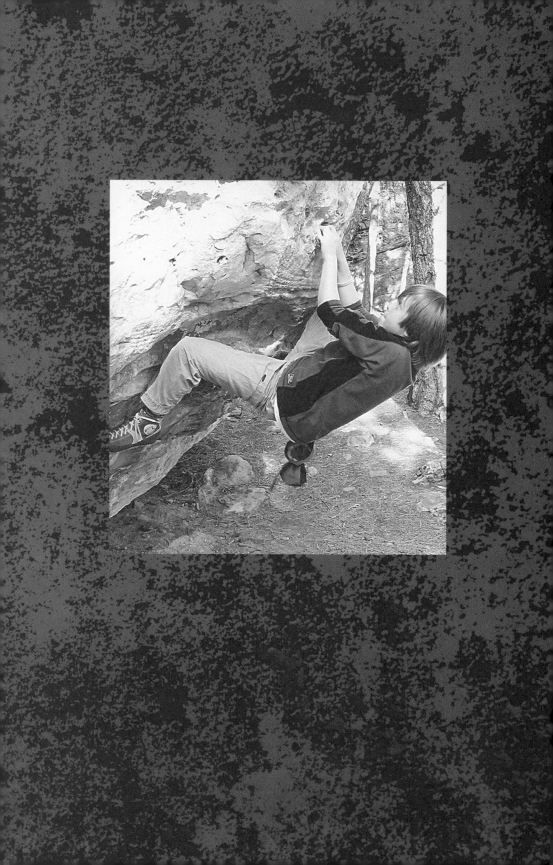

17 Bouldering and Roped Rock Climbing

Sue and I spent our boys' most recent spring break on a rock climbing trip to Joshua Tree National Park in south-central California. Before we left home, we weren't sure how the trip would go. Though Sue and I had climbed quite a bit before the boys were born, neither of us had done much climbing in the years since. Still, the idea of the trip seemed a good one. The boys, at ages 10 and 8, were eager to test their skills beyond the local crags we'd climbed up to that point, and Sue and I long had wanted to see what all the fuss over Joshua Tree was about.

As it turned out, the trip went extremely well. Sue and I learned that we still enjoy climbing—of the safe, top-rope variety as opposed to the traditional, big-wall type I gave up in my 20s. Taylor and Logan loved the immersion into big-time climbing that the trip entailed. And we learned that the fuss over Joshua Tree is well deserved.

More than 4500 climbing routes have been established on the thousands of boulders and cliff faces found throughout the 100,000-acre high-desert park. Those routes and countless others yet to be sent attract hundreds of thousands of climbers to Joshua Tree each year.

Joshua Tree's popularity is due in no small part to its proximity to the Los Angeles metropolitan area. (It's only 140 miles to the west.) It is due as well to the fact that conditions for climbing at Joshua Tree are best in winter, when many climbing sites elsewhere in the country are blanketed in snow. Finally, Joshua Tree is justifiably popular for the sheer magnitude of climbing it affords climbers, all of it on top-quality granite with good edges and plenty of cracks.

The fact that Joshua Tree's crags were busy with climbers made the experience special for the boys. Taylor and Logan were far younger than the 20- to 40-something climbers among whom they climbed, yet the boys felt a kinship and established a solid rapport with their fellow climbers nonetheless.

And though the park was crowded, we had no trouble snagging a campsite 40 feet from a granite face boasting a number of 5.6 and 5.7 friction climbs that provided a perfect challenge for the boys' budding abilities to smear their feet and latch onto nubbins with their fingertips. (For definitions of climbing ratings, see "Ratings," page 186.)

The Basics

■ With the sport of rock climbing, the progression from indoor rock gym to bouldering to top roping to full-on sport or traditional climbing is a logical one to follow with your kids.

■ Manufacturers make special climbing harnesses that enable you to take your kids climbing when they're as young as 3.

■ Bouldering, the newest form of climbing, doesn't even require the use of ropes and harnesses. To give bouldering a try, all you and your kids need are climbing shoes—and even those aren't mandatory.

■ Your kids will see top-rope rock climbing as death-defyingly extreme, yet top roping is as safe as outdoor adventuring gets.

Starting Out

It may not seem like it at first thought, but climbing is one of the easiest and safest outdoor sports to take on with your kids, whether at a climbing mecca like Joshua Tree, or at any local climbing crag or indoor gym. Better yet, as Sue and I have learned with our boys, climbing is

Climbing Types

Want to start a fight? Tell a devotee of traditional, or trad, climbing you think sport climbing is better, or vice versa.

Trad climbing is what most people first picture when they think of rock climbing. It's the process of ascending a rock face by placing protective devices called nuts and cams into cracks in the rock, clipping a rope to those devices for safety, and then climbing on upward. While trad climbing, a lead climber goes first, placing protection along the way, while a belayer feeds out the rope as the lead climber advances. If the lead climber falls, the belayer applies the brakes to the rope and halts the fall. Traditional climbs of such monster walls as Yosemite's Half Dome and El Capitan are what first brought rock climbing to the attention of the general public.

Sport climbing has emerged over the last two decades to challenge trad climbing in popularity. Sport climbers clip into bolts that have been drilled close together into routes up short cliff faces. Sport climbers ascend in great safety from one bolt to the next, clipping the rope to each with metal devices called carabiners. The result? Sport climbers need no training in how to place protective devices, and so are free to attempt extremely difficult moves early on in their climbing careers.

Top roping, which involves running a rope from a belayer to the top of a short face and back down to a climber, is the ultimate form of safe sport climbing. It's also the logical way to introduce your kids to the sport.

Another type of rock climbing is **bouldering**, whereby climbers work to "send" or successfully climb short routes or "problems" on low-level faces that don't require ropes and the placement of protection.

It's worth noting that, much like the sport of gymnastics, many of the best climbers in the world are teenagers because their strength-to-weight ratios are so high. The message for you? If you and your youngsters take up climbing, be prepared for your kids to quickly be able to send routes that are far beyond your ability.

For more general information on rock climbing, visit www.rock-climbing.com. For more information about bouldering, go to www.bouldering.com.

virtually guaranteed to be seen as totally radical by your youngsters.

Climbing, whether roped or unroped, is one of the few "outdoor" action sports you can at first tackle indoors with your kids. It's easy to try climbing at any of the hundreds of rock gyms and climbing walls across the country. Rock gyms (cavernous rooms with fake holds bolted to the walls) and rock walls (popular in community recre-

---

Ratings

Rock climbing routes and bouldering routes are rated for difficulty in different ways.

Climbing routes use the Class 5 portion of the Yosemite Decimal System (see more on page 123) divided into a 1-to-15 scale. Technical rock climbs (those requiring a rope for safety) that are easiest are rated 5.1, and those that are the most difficult are rated 5.15.

A 5.1 route might consist of a roped scramble along an exposed ridge, while a 5.14 or 5.15 route might be up an overhanging face of rock that would appear impossible for mere mortals to climb. Indeed, few adults are capable of climbing routes above 5.11 in difficulty. Mid-level routes of the sort many children are capable of sending fall in the 5.5 and 5.6 range.

Bouldering routes use the still-evolving Vermin Bouldering Scale, with levels of difficulty ranging from V0 to V14. A V0 bouldering route or problem equates roughly to the most difficult move of a 5.9 climb. That means most children will not be able to send bouldering routes tough enough to be rated on the V scale. Instead, when bouldering with your kids, you'll need to look for routes and problems on your own that fit your children's ability levels.

---

ation centers) are located nationwide. To find one near you, go to www.phoenixrockgym.com and click on "Links" for a list of more than 300 rock gyms across the country.

Rock gyms are great places for your kids to hang out with other climbers and be part of the climbing scene, especially during winter months. In addition, your kids will gain confidence and experience by climbing indoors, and that will transfer well to outdoor climbing.

Gym climbing is essentially top roping indoors, and it is equally as safe—minus any danger whatsoever of loose rocks falling from above.

The cost of climbing at a rock gym roughly equates to the cost of using a health club, with yearly, monthly, and daily rates, and lower rates for children. Climbing lessons are generally available.

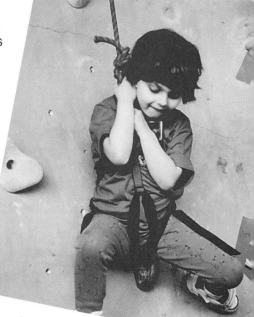

If you and your kids like your indoor introduction to the sport, you can then choose to pursue it outdoors via the logical next step, bouldering. Bouldering—climbing on low-level rock faces and overhangs without ropes—is the newest form of rock climbing. Many bouldering routes don't even involve reaching the top of anything. Rather, a truly extreme bouldering route may require a climber to merely move sideways from one point on a rock face to another, with the climber perhaps no more than a few inches off the ground throughout the entire route.

Bouldering is not so much about the original challenge of big-wall rock climbing—cheating death—as it is about solving climbing "problems" or "puzzles." Gear-wise, bouldering is simple. Boulderers need only climbing shoes for their feet and chalk for their hands. Kids, meanwhile, can get along with tennis shoes and no chalk at all. Many boulderers lay thick foam pads on the ground to cushion their falls, though you'll likely act as the foam pad for your kids when they attempt their rad bouldering moves.

You need never have climbed to take your kids bouldering. A call to your local climbing shop or rock gym will reveal the most popular bouldering spots in your area. Hit the internet to research bouldering possibilities in locations you plan to visit with your kids. Then consider turning to guidebooks for specific route/problem descriptions. Guidebooks to bouldering hot spots are common these days, including, for example, *New England Bouldering* by Tim Kemple (Wolverine Publishing, 2004).

Be prepared for a heavy dose of the hip teen and 20-something scene at any local bouldering hot spots you visit with your kids. Be prepared, as well, to have those same ultra-cool boulderers warmly welcome your kids to their playground, take your kids under wing, and show them the best routes for kids at the site, complete with move demonstrations and spotting help.

FEAR FACTOR?

Jon Ross has been teaching kids to climb on New York's Shawangunk Cliffs for decades. He is quick to point out that, based on his experience, the fearlessness many adults ascribe to children is highly overrated when it comes to rock climbing.

"I've found that children are much more involved in the satisfaction of completing a climb," he says. "It's the achievement, it's taking three, four, five tries and finally getting to the end of a pitch. For children, that's much more powerful than the adrenaline rush of climbing high off the ground."

It's worth noting that climbing isn't for every kid, and may not be for yours. If your children don't like the idea of venturing far up a cliff face, don't push them. There are plenty of other outdoor sports to try with them instead.

"The youngster has to be excited about it or it's no fun for anyone," says Ross.

Rope-rescue-course instructor Leo Lloyd is the father of three young rock climbers in Durango. "Climbing isn't something I've made my kids do," Lloyd says. "I've just offered it to them." As it has turned out, Lloyd's children and others he has taken climbing have picked up the sport with ease.

"Kids are natural climbers," Lloyd says, "and the ones I've taken climbing have just loved the sport."

Lloyd takes his kids top roping regularly. He's now teaching his oldest son, Kendall, 13, to set and remove protection during trad climbs (see "Climbing Types," page 185). Kendall already climbs demanding 5.9 routes and is on track to climb one of the many vertical sandstone towers jutting from the floor of the Utah desert with his father.

Lloyd says that in addition to the fun he has rock climbing with his kids, he appreciates the life lessons climbing teaches them. "When you're climbing, you have to trust whoever's at the other end of the rope," Lloyd says. "And you have to trust yourself. You have to find it within yourself to make a tough move. That trust—of yourself as well as others—relates directly to life."

Ross says the fearlessness many adults ascribe to children is highly overrated when it comes to rock climbing.

Moving On Up

When presented with the possibility of going rock climbing, most kids picture using ropes and ascending to great, scary heights. If you're to pursue climbing with your kids for long, you'll likely need to deliver on that expectation.

I first took Taylor, then 6, and Logan, then 3, roped rock climbing with a friend and his two children. We set up a top rope at a local climbing face. Up the kids went one by one, tethered to the rope by a children's climbing harness.

Adults climbing on either side of our party offered the four kids loads of encouragement. In response, the kids, a little nervous at the outset of the adventure, became fearless. They scrambled up the cliff like tennis-shoed monkeys, worked their way back and forth across the face to try different holds and more challenging routes, and swung far out from the rock when my friend or I lowered them to the ground.

The entire experience was pure fun for the kids. Moreover, though they thought of what they were doing as death-defyingly extreme, they in fact were far safer tied in to the top rope than they would have been playing on playground equipment unroped.

In the years since, Taylor and Logan have found little excitement in climbing on the line-up-and-wait-your-turn indoor rock wall at our local community recreation center. They love the freedom of the outdoor climbing and bouldering we continue to do on faces around town, however. And they had an absolute blast at Joshua Tree.

If you've climbed yourself or can latch on to a kid-friendly climber, it's easy to go out to a local face and set up a top rope for your kids to monkey around on. If you're starting from scratch, it's equally easy to sign up for any of the many family rock climbing courses offered by climbing schools and guide services nationwide.

Outdoor climbing areas are found near virtually every city in the country these days. To locate those near you, cruise the internet or call your local climbing shop or outdoor retailer.

To get a taste of the climbing and bouldering worlds in general, check out www.climbing.com, www.bouldering.com, and, if you're in the Northeast, www.newenglandbouldering.com.

Climbing Gear for Kids

An easy way to get your youngsters excited about the idea of rock climbing is to surprise them with their very own **chalk bags**. (Rock jocks use chalk from these small nylon bags, slung around their waists, to make their sweaty hands less slippery as they climb.) Your little-kid rock jocks will love the idea that you consider them ready for such big-kid climbing accoutrements—and they may be more likely to take to climbing as a result.

Tennis shoes are fine for beginning kid climbers. If your kids like either bouldering or roped climbing, however, they'll quickly benefit from the added traction true **climbing shoes** provide. Specifically for kid climbers, EB (www.eb-france.com) makes the Baboon and the New Monkey climbing shoe models, Montrail (www.montrail.com) makes the Grommet and Grommet Girl, and Five.Ten (www.fiveten.com) offers the Velcro. The multicolored Velcro is made of recycled scrap leather, something your enviro kids may find cool.

If your kids are going to do much more than low-level bouldering, they'll need **helmets** designed specifically for climbing. The German climbing gear manufacturer Edelrid (www.edelrid.de) makes the Ultralight Jr. for kids. The helmet, a small version of the popular Ultralight, is designed to fit children up to age 14 and is available through a number of climbing gear retailers, including REI (www.rei.com).

Finally, kids up to 80 pounds need the added safety a children's **harness** gives them. The full-body kids' harness made by Trango (www.trango.com) is designed for children weighing 25 to 80 pounds. After that, kids' hips are developed enough to accommodate an adult-style harness that straps around the waist but not the upper body. Black Diamond (www.bdel.com) makes two around-the-waist harnesses for kids that are recommended only for top roping. The company says its kids' harnesses are for children ages 5 to 10.

Possibilities

JOSHUA TREE NATIONAL PARK

Bouldering and roped climbing hot spots exist across the country, and the one that is known to everyone is Joshua Tree National Park in south-central California.

Will Joshua Tree be crowded with climbers if you decide to show up there with your kids during the not-too-hot fall/winter/spring months? Assuredly. But will being part of that climbing scene get your kids excited about taking on a sport that is all about extreme fun and radical adventure? No doubt it will.

Camping is available in the park's several campgrounds, including the most popular among climbers, Hidden Valley. Also, hotel/motel accommodations are available just outside the park. For more information about Joshua Tree, visit www.nps.gov/jotr.

In many cases, kids are exposed to climbing through their schools, Scouts, and indoor gyms, and they drag their parents out to try the sport.

MUIR VALLEY

Tech-publishing magnate and rock climbing philanthropist Rick Weber and his wife, Liz, have purchased and created a one-of-a-kind preserve for rock climbing and nature walking in rural eastern Kentucky that is perfect for family climbing excursions.

The 400-acre Muir Valley is walled by 7 miles of hard sandstone cliffs that offer a wide range of sport climbs. Since the preserve's establishment in 2004, volunteers have placed hundreds of bolted climbs on the cliffs that ring the valley. The cliffs average 50 feet in height, perfect for top roping.

Access to the valley, already extremely popular with families, is free. Go to www.muirvalley.com for more information.

HIGH ANGLE ADVENTURES AND THE GUNKS

An hour and a half north of New York City, near New Paltz, New York, the Shawangunk Cliffs, or the Gunks, have been a climbing mecca for decades. Jon Ross, owner of High Angle Adventures, has been a fixture there for just as long.

Ross, who has been climbing since 1958, founded High Angle Adventures in 1974. He and his team of guides offer private classes geared specifically to their clients, be they adults, children, or families. Because of the personal, one-on-one nature of High Angle's guide service, Ross doesn't set a minimum age limit on the children he and his instructors teach.

"I've taught children as young as 5," he says. "But age isn't the factor I'm worried about. I'm looking for parents who say, 'I can't keep this kid on the ground. Every time I turn around, he's at the top of the jungle gym or up a tree.'"

Ross says more and more kids and families are showing up at the Gunks these days.

"Kids are exposed to climbing through their schools, Scouts, and indoor climbing gyms," he explains. In many cases, Ross reports, it's the kids who are dragging their parents out to learn rock climbing rather than the other way around.

The result?

"It's enormously satisfying for everyone involved," Ross says. "But the kids, especially, just love it."

High Angle Adventures' private, daylong courses are $125 per person with four people per guide. For more information about High Angle, call 800-777-2546 or visit www.highangle.com.

193

EMS CLIMBING SCHOOL FAMILY PROGRAM

The outdoor retailer Eastern Mountain Sports' Climbing School runs a half-day introduction-to-rock-climbing course for families in five locations in the Northeast: North Conway, New Hampshire; Rumney, New Hampshire; Lake Placid, New York; New Paltz, New York (the Gunks); and on crags in the greater Boston area.

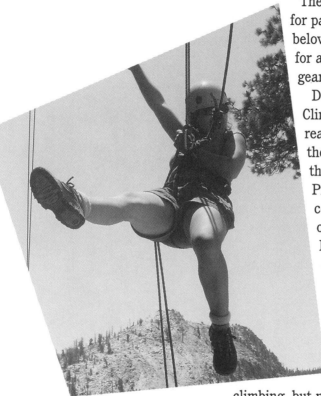

The course, designed for parents with children below age 12, costs $300 for a family of four. All gear is provided.

David Kelly, EMS Climbing School's outreach manager, says the difference between the EMS Family Program and other courses the school offers is that the Family Program is designed to be experiential as opposed to overly instructional. "During the course, we teach parents and kids the basics of climbing, but not necessarily a lot of technical skills," says Kelly. "The idea is to get the kids and parents off the ground and climbing. We try to make it relatively easy for kids so they have fun and are successful."

For more information about the program, call 800-310-4504 or visit www.emsclimb.com.

MOUNTAIN ADVENTURE SEMINARS

Bear Valley, California-based Mountain Adventure Seminars offers what may well be the most affordable outdoor action sport clinic in the country.

Each summer, Mountain Adventure owners Kimi and Aaron Johnson offer a full-day Family Rock Climbing Program for $50 per person ($45 for REI members). The introductory program, which includes all gear, is run at four northern California locations: two in the San Francisco Bay area, one near Sacramento, and one at Mountain Adventure's headquarters in Bear Valley, three and a half hours east of the Bay Area in the central Sierra.

"We're trying to make it affordable," says Kimi Johnson of the discounted introductory program. "We hope kids and moms and dads will like it and come back to do more with us."

For more information about the program, call 209-753-6556 or visit www.mtadventure.com.

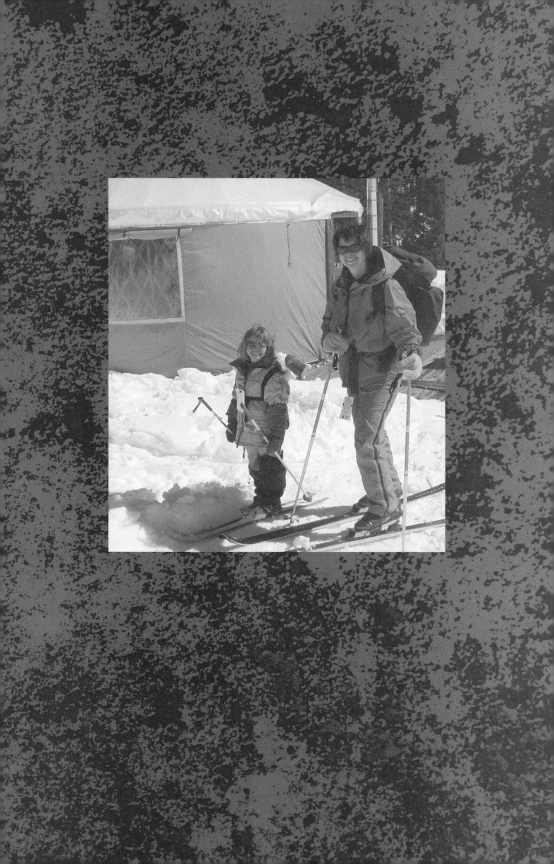

18 Backcountry Skiing

Backcountry skiing is one sport that doesn't immediately leap to mind when considering outdoor sports to try with kids. You may find the sport worth exploring, however, because it offers you and your kids the opportunity to get outdoors and into the backcountry together in winter. It does require, however, that you have access to snow-covered hills and mountains, and that you are schooled in avalanche and winter safety.

You may not want to try backcountry skiing with your kids when they're youngsters, but older kids, starting at age 9 or 10, have the coordination and strength necessary to ski in the backcountry, assuming you head up established ski trails or do the trail breaking yourself.

In backcountry skiing, the binding attaches only the toe to the ski, allowing the heel to travel up and down as skiers stride up snow-covered slopes or peaks or across snow-covered meadows. There are three styles of backcountry skiing:

■ Nordic skiing involves lightweight gear that enables the skier to move quickly along tracks in snow that in many cases are already broken. Nordic skiers often use special wax on the bottom of their skis that allows their skis to glide speedily through the snow.

■ Telemark skiers use beefier skis with climbing skins, synthetic strips that stick to the bottom of the skis and prevent skiers from sliding backward as they climb. They typically "break" a new trail upward through the snow, then remove their climbing skins from their skis to free-heel ski downward in a distinctive bent-knee crouch.

■ Alpine touring involves the use of downhill-style equipment with a special heel binding that releases for uphill striding, then locks into place for traditional alpine skiing.

Of the three backcountry skiing styles, telemarking is the most fun to pursue with kids—though that has become true only recently, with the appearance on the market of kid-specific telemark gear.

Nordic skis are too lightweight to be skied downhill easily, which is the part of backcountry skiing kids love. Heavy alpine-touring skis, boots, and bindings, meanwhile, are designed for mountaineering-style skiing that requires more strength and stamina than preadolescents possess.

Telemark skiing falls between Nordic skiing and alpine touring. The new kids' telemark gear is light enough for children to stride uphill in the backcountry, yet heavy enough to provide stability for them to free-heel ski down whatever slopes they ascend. As a result, the sport now lends itself well to preadolescent thrill seekers.

Telemark skiing is enjoying a tremendous boom among teens and adults across the country. The number of telemark skiers in America has increased more than 200 percent over the last few years, and more than 300 percent among 16- to 24-year-olds.

The Basics

■ Among the several forms of backcountry skiing, telemarking makes the most sense to try with your kids.

■ In response to the telemark skiing boom, gear manufacturers are just beginning to introduce kid-size telemark gear.

■ Safety through avalanche-zone avoidance is paramount when it comes to taking your kids into the backcountry in winter.

■ Multiday ski trips to backcountry yurts and cabins are entirely possible and loads of fun with kids.

Getting Started

Sue and I jumped into telemark skiing during an earlier boom the sport enjoyed in the 1980s. Back then, telemark skiing was just evolving from Nordic skiing to become its own sport—albeit a sport similar to the earliest style of free-heel skiing practiced in Scandinavia as far back as the 16th century. In the 1980s, telemark gear consisted of leather boots, lightweight bindings, and metal-edged skis only slightly sturdier than Nordic-specific gear. Since then, telemark gear has evolved until it more closely resembles downhill ski gear than Nordic gear. Today's telemark boots are plastic, bindings are heavy duty, and skis are essentially interchangeable with downhill skis.

As a result of new, kid-specific gear, telemark skiing now lends itself well to preadolescent thrill seekers.

Sue and I telemarked throughout the two decades of the telemark gear revolution. For most of that time, we skied only in the backcountry, where we enjoyed long days of sun and swooping lines through deep powder.

Then we had kids. We stuck with skiing in the backcountry with Taylor and Logan in backpacks for as long as we could, though what formerly had been days of steep climbs followed by downhill descents became, instead, sedate backcountry tours on level trails.

Soon enough, our boys grew too big for us to carry into the backcountry. But they were nowhere near old enough to ski the backcountry on their own, or to handle the challenge of downhill skiing on telemark skis.

What to do?

Just emerging from their toddler years, the boys were old enough to begin either Nordic skiing or fixed-heel downhill skiing. If Sue and I wanted to continue to ski together with Taylor and Logan as a family, we had two choices. We could go to a groomed Nordic ski center and kick and glide with the boys on tiny Nordic skis. Or we could go to a lift-assisted downhill area and telemark ski while the boys downhilled on tiny fixed-heel skis.

STARTING OUT AT A DOWNHILL AREA

My family chose the raucous, music-blasting world of our local downhill area over the quiet serenity of the local Nordic center just across the highway. Sue and I were

addicted to the downhill rush of telemarking, so while we
continued telemarking, Taylor and Logan became miniature downhillers. Over time, more and more telemarkers,
part of today's boom, joined us on the slopes of our local
downhill area.

As with introducing climbing to your children at an
indoor rock gym, a good way to get your kids ready for
the backcountry is to pick up some telemark gear for
them and first begin telemark skiing with them at a
downhill area. Skiing down a mountain with free heels
isn't easy. But it's far easier on groomed snow than
in deep powder. (The challenge
with starting
your kids tele-
marking at a ski
resort first is tear-
ing them away
from the easily
gained vertical of a
lift-served area to
slog uphill in the back-
country with you. Still,
taking non-telemark-ski-
ing youngsters straight
into the backcountry is
extremely challenging, if
not impossible.)

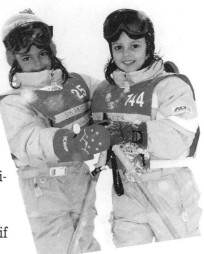

Thanks to the boom in
telemark skiing, many ski resorts and associated rental
shops carry rental telemark gear for kids. For now, the
telemark boom is bigger in the West than in the East.
That means kid telemark gear is more widely available to
rent at resorts in the Rockies and Sierra than in the
Northeast. Time will tell if the telemark boom continues
and expands. In the meantime, check ahead rather than
assume any resort you choose to visit will have kid telemark gear available for rent.

Some resorts now offer child-only telemark clinics.
Beaver Creek Resort (www.beavercreek.com), west of
Denver in central Colorado, is one. You can also hire a

Telemark Gear for Kids

When it comes to gear, telemark skiing is just opening up to children. Whether the kid market for telemark gear will continue to grow depends on how popular kid telemarking becomes in the years ahead. In the meantime, Karhu (www.karhu.com) and K2 (www.k2skis.com) make kid-specific **telemark skis**. Karhu's ski, the Special Agent, comes complete with attention-grabbing, James Bond-style graphics. In addition, short adult skis work perfectly well as kid telemark skis. The Karhu skis come in three sizes, 123 centimeter, 133 centimeter, and 143 centimeter, making them suitable for kids from ages 6 or 7 to 12 or 13.

Garmont (www.garmont.com) makes the bright orange Teledactyl, the only kid **telemark boot** on the market. Since its introduction, the boot has become virtually essential equipment for kid telemark skiers. The Teledactyl is made of pliable plastic that is soft enough to flex when children execute their crouched telemark turns.

You and your kids will need skins that attach to ski bottoms for the uphill climbing you'll do in the backcountry. **Climbing skins** feature nylon hairs that point backward, grabbing the snow and providing traction when weighted, and sliding forward easily when unweighted. Though strap-on skins are available, most backcountry skiers use skins that stick to the bottoms of their skis because the superior traction of such skins makes them less likely to slip on steep slopes. Three manufacturers make adhesive climbing skins: Black Diamond (www.bdel.com), Backcountry Access (www.bcaccess.com), and G3 (www.genuineguidegear.com).

Kids are light enough that only half a skin stuck under each of their skis provides adequate traction for climbing uphill. That means one pair of skins (with each skin cut in half) will service two pairs of kids' skis.

For great information about telemark gear and telemark skiing in general, visit online telemark gear retailer www.telemarkski.com.

telemark instructor at a resort to provide a clinic for your whole family.

STARTING OUT AT A NORDIC CENTER

There's one big plus in getting your kids prepared for the backcountry by starting them at a Nordic center: It'll be much easier to coax your kids from the flat trails to head into the hills for some downhill telemarking than to convince them to leave a lift-served area behind.

Once your kids are comfortable with the free-heel aspect of Nordic skiing, they'll make the switch to free-heel telemark skiing with ease.

Steep Learning Curves

At age 9, after six years of alpine skiing at a downhill resort, Taylor surprised us when he asked if he could try telemarking. A couple of his friends had taken up the sport at the behest of their telemarker parents, and he wanted to see what it was all about.

Logic says Sue and I should have jumped at the opportunity to turn Taylor on to "our" sport. But we hesitated. Telemark skiing demands far more balance than fixed-heel downhill skiing and so can be frustrating to anyone trying to learn it—especially someone who has yet to turn 10.

Taylor kept hounding us, however. He telemarked with a friend's gear for a couple of days and professed to love the sport. Sue and I talked. If Taylor was willing to buy telemark skis with his own money, we told him, we'd pitch in for his boots.

It would help the premise of this book if I could report that today Taylor has become a telemark skiing fiend. But that hasn't been the case. Instead, he has gone back and forth between fixed-heel and free-heel skiing since he got his telemark gear. He likes both, but acknowledges the challenges telemarking presents.

Nonetheless, Taylor's foray into telemark skiing has presented a great opportunity to our family. Now that he's telemarking—no matter how rudimentarily—Taylor is set to head into the backcountry on skis. That prospect has him and Sue and me excited. Sue and I have yet to head

"The kids never want to leave," says Jeanne Pastore of her family's backcountry yurt ski trips.

into the backcountry with Taylor, however, because we're waiting (anxiously) for Logan to be able to join us. As soon as he's old enough to do so, away we'll go. In the meantime, however, we know plenty of folks who regularly ski the backcountry with their kids.

Our friends Jeanne and Mark Pastore and their children, Alicia Rose, 12, and Gino, 10, for example, take a multiday ski trip to a backcountry yurt every winter. "The kids absolutely love it," says Jeanne of the family's annual winter getaway. "It's similar to backpacking except it's all snow play."

On their backcountry trips, the Pastores pull a sled filled with gear. By staying in a yurt with a wood stove, Alicia Rose and Gino can play and get wet and cold in the snow all day long, and then dry their clothes and warm themselves indoors off and on during the day and throughout the evening.

"The kids never want to leave," Jeanne adds. "The family bonding we do is just incredible. There are no distractions, no schedules. It's just us."

Jeanne also appreciates the reminder the family's annual yurt trips provide of just how simple life can be. "We live just fine on next to nothing—a wood stove for heat, some

203

Variations on a Backcountry Theme

A look at backcountry snow sports other than telemark skiing:

Nordic

Backcountry Nordic skiing, off groomed trails, is a fine, away-from-it-all pastime you and your kids are likely to enjoy together. Nordic skiing with your kids at a Nordic center with groomed trails, though not a full-on backcountry experience, is a truly good kid experience as well.

The groomed-trail nature of Nordic skiing lends itself far better to young children (up to age 10 or so) than does backcountry telemark skiing. As a precursor to backcountry telemarking, you may prefer to start your kids out Nordic skiing at a Nordic center to starting them out fixed-heel downhill skiing (or telemarking) at a downhill area.

Alpine Touring

Alpine touring (AT) is, generally speaking, as extreme as backcountry skiing gets. AT equipment is a cross between telemark and downhill ski gear. The heels of AT bindings release to allow the skier to stride up a slope. The heels then lock into place when the skier is ready to ski back down the mountain. As a result, an alpine tourer skis the same as a fixed-heel downhiller, enabling the tourer to attempt more challenging descents than most telemark skiers. No AT gear manufacturers make gear designed for children.

Snowboarding

Snowboarding is the backcountry winter sport of choice for many teens and 20-somethings. Most of those who snowboard in the "backcountry" do so simply by riding out of bounds at resorts or by hiking a short distance from a road and building jumps or ramps to play on.

Some boarders strap snowboards to their backs and hike, snowshoe, or climb far from roads to take lengthy rides down long slopes or off the summits of mountains. Such true backcountry adventures are both fun and extreme, but preadolescents can't handle the demanding uphill climbs such excursions require, no matter how capable of snowboarding back down a backcountry route they may be.

food, and a few pots for melting snow and cooking," she says. "It's good to be reminded that you don't really need anything more than that to be happy."

The Pastores do plenty of day ski trips into the backcountry as well. "With skins on their telemark skis, the kids can go anywhere," Jeanne says.

But the family doesn't, in fact, go just anywhere. When it comes to avalanche danger, they are extremely cautious. Before Alicia Rose and Gino were born, Jeanne and Mark toured and telemarked avalanche terrain while wearing avalanche beacons. Nowadays, with the kids, says Jeanne, "If we need beacons to go someplace, we just don't go there."

Instead, the Pastores stick to slopes that don't present avalanche danger. They choose the yurts they stay in based on the same criteria.

All concessionaires of winter backcountry yurts and cabins provide maps that note nearby avalanche-danger zones. "We use those maps to know where we can ski safely with our kids, and we stick to those areas," says Jeanne. "We also use all our avalanche-safety knowledge to be sure we're always in safe areas with our kids."

Over the years, the Pastores have known several friends and acquaintances who have been caught or killed in avalanches, and Sue and I have friends who have encountered avalanches as well. There's simply no point in exposing children to such dangers.

Before you head into the backcountry, ask around at local ski and outdoor shops for advice on where to head into the backcountry with your kids in your area. Start with locations that are popular with other backcountry enthusiasts so that your kids are among other skiers, even if most will be adults.

As with snowshoeing, choose sunny, warm days for heading into the backcountry with your kids. Remember, backcountry skiing will be much tougher for your kids than it will be for you because the ratio of the weight of your kids' ski gear to their body weight will be significantly higher than the weight of your gear to your body weight. Plan accordingly by keeping your excursions short and spiced with lots of treats.

Ask local ski and outdoor shops about the best places to take kids into the backcountry.

You will also have to get up to speed on avalanche danger and safety, preferably through one of the many avalanche-awareness courses offered in snow country each winter. Go to www.avalanche.org for a list of courses by region.

Possibilities

SKI HUTS

Turning yourself and your kids into backcountry skiers opens your family to the big wide world of ski-hut trips. Backcountry cabins and yurts, universally known as huts, are available for rental throughout snow country.

Some such cabins have electricity; many don't. Some have running water; many don't. Some are located deep in the backcountry; many more are located an easy ski in from the nearest plowed road.

Serious skiers undertake epic backcountry hut-to-hut trips that are several days in length. With your kids, you'll likely prefer skiing to one close-to-the-road hut and using it as a base for a night or two—though even a trip of that sort won't be easy. You'll be faced with carrying food, bedding, emergency supplies, and plenty of warm clothing on your back or in a sled while skiing into the backcountry, where weather and avalanche safety will be concerns. Still, as noted earlier in this chapter, many families love the hut trips they take each winter.

In addition to the huts described in this section, search "ski huts" on the internet for lists of huts by state that interest you, then narrow your search from there.

PORTNEUF RANGE YURT SYSTEM

The Portneuf Range Yurt System is composed of five yurts in the Portneuf Mountains southeast of Pocatello in southeastern Idaho, two hours north of Salt Lake City. The Portneuf range is known for light powder snow and outstanding backcountry skiing. Each yurt is outfitted with pots, an ax, bunk beds, a wood stove for heat, a gas stove for cooking, and a gas lantern for light. The yurts are spaced to accommodate multiday yurt-to-yurt trips, though you'll likely prefer using a single yurt as a base for your family. Three of the five yurts are accessible by children and families.

The Portneuf yurts are operated by volunteers in cooperation with the Idaho State University Outdoor Program. Advance reservations are required. Rates range from $40 to $70 per yurt per night, depending on yurt size and whether you rent on a weekday or a weekend. For more information, call 208-282-2945 or visit www.isu.edu/outdoor (keyword: yurts).

SIERRA CLUB HUTS

The Sierra Club owns and operates four backcountry cabins in the Lake Tahoe area of the Sierra high country near the Nevada border in California. The huts are extremely popular with backcountry skiers, and reservations far in advance are required.

One of the greatest things about these huts, to kids and adults alike, is that enough snow falls during some winters to bury the two-story cabins, requiring visitors to access them via tunnels and/or upper-story doorways.

The huts are located an average of 3 miles from the nearest plowed road—a doable distance for children age 9 or so and up.

Each hut sleeps 12 to 15 people. For more information, call 800-679-6775 or visit www.sierraclub.org (keyword: huts).

10TH MOUNTAIN DIVISION HUTS

The same cabins for summer hut-to-hut hiking in Colorado are premier winter backcountry ski cabins as well. The most accessible of the cabins are as popular in winter as they are in summer; reservations are essential. If you plan to ski to them with kids, you'll have to choose with care those cabins for which access doesn't involve avalanche danger.

For an overview of the 10th Mountain Division huts, see page 168. For detailed information, call 970-925-5775 or visit www.huts.org.

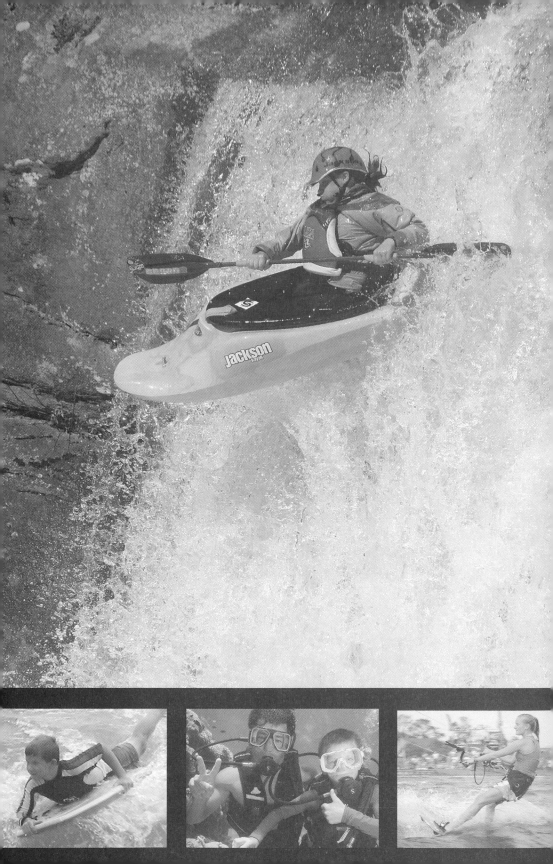

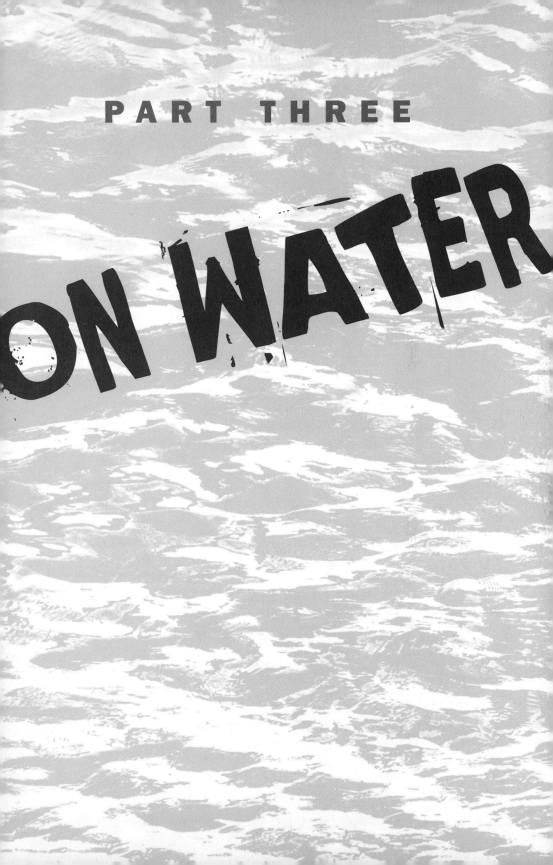

PART THREE

ON WATER

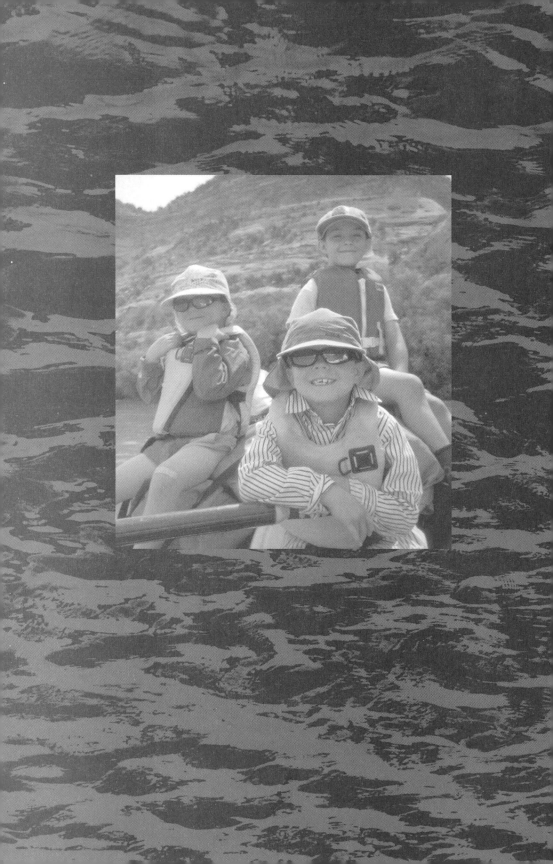

19 River Running

Sue and I applied for a permit to float the San Juan River through the redrock country of southeastern Utah when Taylor was 4 and Logan 1. Our 56-mile trip through the desert wilderness, scheduled for July, should have been a relaxing, low-water journey well after the end of spring runoff. Instead, thunderstorms in the days leading up to our departure turned the San Juan into a raging torrent—and made our first-ever river trip far more extreme than we'd envisioned.

The clouds disappeared the day before our trip commenced. We set off in our rented raft beneath cobalt skies. Instantly, the river took control, shooting us downstream at the roller-coaster-like speed of 8 miles per hour instead of the usual July low-water speed of 2 to 3 miles per hour. When I first attempted to put our raft ashore, the craft bounced off the beach and spun crazily back into the main current. (My inability to land our boat wasn't helped by the fact that I'd never before rowed a raft or any other water craft—something I probably shouldn't be confessing in these pages.)

As day one wore on, Sue and I learned to beach the raft despite the ripping current. We also learned to float downstream sideways, ready to pull or push on the oars and straighten the boat to avoid oncoming rocks. And we learned to row upstream, against the current, when necessary to slow our descent and provide us more time to choose our route down the river.

Three days into the trip, Sue and the boys walked around the only Class III rapid on the stretch of river we were running. I rowed through it, successfully avoiding a hole on the left side of the river that appeared, to my inexperienced eyes, capable of swallowing a Mack truck.

The ferocity of the current was such that, even onshore, Sue and I did not allow Taylor and Logan to remove their personal floatation devices, except when they were inside the tent. In addition, Sue and I each took responsibility for one of the boys while we were onshore, never letting our assigned charges wander from our sight.

The Basics

- A river trip has all the necessary elements for an ideal kid trip—sand, mud, water, motion, adventure, exploration, and, hopefully, sun.

- The number of river miles run each day doesn't matter to kids; the amount of fun they have does.

- Terrific possibilities for family river running adventures—day excursions and multiday trips alike—exist in every region of the country.

With our more experienced rafting family companions, we camped at the mouth of Grand Gulch our last night on the river. Thanks to the thunderstorms that preceded our trip, the side canyon gushed with red muddy water as thick as pea soup. We played in the Gulch's sun-warmed stream and climbed behind waterfalls to peer out through flooding curtains cascading over rock ledges.

By the time we oared the final stretch of flatwater to the takeout the next day, Sue and I were addicted to the fun and adventurousness of family river running. In the years since, we've continued to run the San Juan regularly, and we've graduated to other rivers of greater degrees of difficulty.

Taylor and Logan began running the San Juan in their own kid-size hard-shell kayaks when each reached the age of 6. When the boys took to the water in their own craft, Sue and I switched from rental rafts to a pair of two-man inflatable kayaks, miniature rafts shaped like fat canoes and maneuvered with sea kayak paddles (see photo on page 232). On our river trips these days, Sue and I paddle our inflatables, also called duckies, as solo crafts, with the excess space in each taken up by our camping gear, while Taylor and Logan spin circles around us in their hard shells.

Family River-Tripping

Sue and I are not alone as family river running addicts. On every river we run, we see other families and groups of families in ever-shifting flotillas of rafts, canoes, hard-shell kayaks, and duckies, lining up for rapids, then spreading amoeba-like across the river again, group members jumping into the water for swims, rafts creeping up on one another to engage in water fights, and kids in kayaks skittering like water bugs among the larger boats.

"A river trip has all the necessary elements for an ideal kid trip—sand, mud, water, motion, adventure, exploration, and, hopefully, sun," says Suzanne Strazza, a former river guide and Outward Bound instructor turned at-home mom. Strazza and her husband have been taking their two sons on rivers since the boys were babies.

Strazza says she and her husband, also a former Outward Bound instructor, have seen firsthand the self-reliance and confidence their boys have developed as a result of the many days they've spent on rivers around the West. "Both of us know the value of being part of a group in a demanding and, at times, unforgiving environment," Strazza says. "Family river trips are like Outward Bound courses for all of us."

Though the river trips Strazza takes with her husband and kids are first and foremost fun, she says she believes the demands the trips invariably place on every member of the family are worthwhile as well.

"I'm convinced the bonds we've forged through our shared adventures will help us withstand the tests that are sure to come as our boys grow up," Strazza says.

How to Have Happy
River Trips with Kids

Go Short

The number of miles run each day doesn't matter to young-sters; the amount of fun they have does.

When Taylor and Logan were very young, Sue and I once spent an entire week "running" (to use the term very loosely) a single 26-mile stretch of the San Juan River in Utah with two other families. All of the parents looked at our slow journey downstream as a car-camping trip without cars—an opportunity to play with our kids on our own private beaches day after day after day. Each time we broke camp and took to the river, our only goal was to make it far enough downstream to be out of sight of the camp we'd just left. Beyond that, we stopped when-ever and wherever something struck our fancy.

Now that Taylor and Logan are piloting their own kayaks, we put in more river miles than when they were little, but we still spend far more time playing and relaxing in camp than most adult-only groups. The result is happy children and content par-ents—the perfect river-trip combination.

Don't Overreach

Don't succumb to the temptation to run a river with rapids that you foresee as too challenging. That may well scare your kids and turn them off river running before they even get the chance to experience the sport.

Start small and work your way up. When your kids are little, the rapids will be for you, not them. When your kids are older, carefully consider what you believe they're ready for.

Let the River Provide the Toys

Beyond a bucket and digging tools for beach play, you don't need to provide toys for your kids on river trips. With beaches, rocks, forests, side canyons, cliffs, and swimming-hole eddies, mul-tiday river trips are one big, toy-free play experience for children.

Keep Treats on Board

Use treats liberally to keep your youngsters happy during the parts of a rafting trip kids find most boring—the flatwater por-tions. (Kids love rapids, provided they're not too big.)

A Nation of Rivers

River journeying has been an integral part of the American experience since man first came to the North American continent. These days, as highways and jets speed us wherever we want to go (except during rush hour and peak holiday flying periods, that is), there's something mystical about floating down a river into the wilderness and into our country's past. That mystique is something your kids will sense the instant you launch on your first river trip with them—the fascination with what's around the next bend, with what adventures await in the river hours or river days ahead.

Terrific possibilities for family river running adventures—day excursions and multiday trips alike—exist in every region of the country. In deciding where and how to undertake a family river trip, you'll be faced with several decisions:

- Whether to go with a guided group or do the trip yourself.

- Whether to go far from home or find something close by.

- What type of boat to use.

- What type of water to run.

Let's look at these decisions one at a time.

GUIDED VS. DO-IT-YOURSELF

There's a lot to be said for first trying out river running with an outfitter. The trade-off, of course, is price. Outfitted and guided river trips don't come cheap. But all the gear you need is provided for you, and safety concerns are taken care of. You and your kids need only clamber aboard and have a great time.

By way of outfitted trips, you can jump on an oared raft for a half-day or day trip, either on a weekend close to home or as part of a vacation. As a step up from that, you can do a half-day or day trip on a paddle raft—one on which the passengers actually paddle the boat based on the guide's commands. As a further step up, you can take a multiday river trip on any number of rivers in the East and West that will present whatever degree of challenge you want.

> There's something mystical about floating with your kids down a river into the wilderness and into our country's past.

215

If you and your kids enjoy any or all such river running possibilities you sample, you may want to undertake a river trip on your own. Such trips aren't as daunting as they may at first seem. You'll be best off starting with day trips, then graduating to multiday trips. (In other words, don't do as Sue and I did and set off first thing on a multiday trip—unless, like us, you do so with an experienced river rafting family or two.)

After day tripping, you'll be ready for a do-it-yourself multiday river trip. You'll be best off teaming up with at least one other family for your inaugural multiday trip; there's safety and comfort in numbers.

NEAR OR FAR

It makes sense to at first try river running close to home. If you like the sport, you can venture farther and more expensively afield.

> **Do-it-yourself river trips aren't as daunting as they may at first seem.**

If you don't foresee a lot of family river running in your future, however, you may want to invest in big-name, big-fun rivers from the get go: the Rogue River in Oregon, the Middle Fork of the Salmon in Idaho, Lodore Canyon of the upper Green River in Colorado, the Chattooga River in South Carolina, or the New River Gorge or Upper Gauley River in West Virginia.

Don't be afraid to leap into river running by signing up first thing for an outfitted multiday trip on a river far from your home. By their very nature, outfitted family river trips, with gear and food provided and safety built in, are as close to a guaranteed adventurous good time for you and your kids as exists in the world of outdoor sports. Provided you have a modicum of car-camping experience, odds are you won't go wrong on any outfitted trip you choose.

Cruise the internet to find rivers that interest you. Even if you're considering do-it-yourself trips, the easiest way to compare potential rivers is to surf outfitted-trip sites. You'll be amazed how many rivers are out there waiting for you.

Note that many rivers require permits for which do-it-yourselfers must apply, often months in advance. In many cases, limited numbers of private-party permits are then allocated via lotteries. If you'll be doing a trip yourself, use the internet to learn how to get a permit and set up your trip.

Never run a river on your own without the best guidebook available for the stretch you'll be running.

BOAT CHOICES

Choosing a means of conveyance for family river trips is as complex as choosing a car. On the road, do you want a sedan, a mini-van, or an SUV? On the water, do you want a bathtub-style raft, a cataraft, or an inflatable kayak? As with cars, each boat type has its pros and cons, depending on your tastes and the difficulty level (see "Whitewater Ratings," page 218) of the rivers you plan to run. (On out-fitted river trips, of course, boat choices will be made for you.)

Inflatable kayaks: Fine for Class I, II, and III rapids, but challenging in Class IV water and dangerous in Class V water.

Pros: Small and light, easy to store, great for do-it-your-selfers (just jump in and start paddling), limited gear-hauling space means you take only what you need, lots of fun in whitewater up to Class III and low Class IV, usually paddled as a solo craft (you get to be master and commander of your own vessel), younger kids love riding up front and getting splashed by waves, increasingly available for rent.

Cons: Limited gear-hauling space, prone to flip in big water (especially when lightly loaded), too small and tippy for Class V water.

Bathtub-style rafts: Fine through Class V water.

Pros: Easy to rent, easy and cheap to buy used, stable, great for babies and toddlers (front passenger well serves as a built-in playpen), lots of room for gear.

Cons: Big and bulky, take up lots of garage storage space, require trailer or pickup bed for transport, heavy (can trash your back!).

Catarafts: Catarafts consist of two inflatable tubes connected by an aluminum frame. They, as well as large, bathtub-style rafts, will take you down everything up to and including the Class V+ rapids of the Grand Canyon.

Whitewater Ratings

River rapids are rated by roman numerals on a I to V scale:

Class I: A few riffles and waves no more than 12 inches high.

Class II: Waves up to 3 feet with a clear line of attack, though some maneuvering is required.

Class III: The fun begins. High, irregular waves, tight passages, extensive and often complex maneuvering. Generally worth scouting.

Class IV: Wicked fun for kids ages 10 and up, depending on means of transport (outfitters often limit rapids of Class IV and up to teenagers). Lengthy, turbulent rapids with many rocks and drops up to 5 feet. Standing waves as high as 6 feet below rapids.

Class V: Over the top. Extremely challenging rapids with difficult routes. Big drops and huge standing waves. Numerous keeper holes and whirlpools.

Note: All moving water is dangerous. People can and do die in Class I water, just as they do in Class V water. There's no substitute for knowledge and preparedness gained through guided trips, river running courses, and a gradual progression from less to more challenging water.

Pros: Highly maneuverable, can haul lots of gear, extremely stable in big water, good seating for kids ages 6 and up, take up less garage storage space (with nesting frame pieces and rolled up tubes), come apart in pieces (resulting in less potential for back strain), frame pieces can be configured in different ways depending on the trip and type of water expected.

Cons: Not as widely available for rent or for sale used, no front passenger well as a playpen for babies and toddlers, require more set-up time.

To learn more about each of these types of boats, visit various online river gear retailers, such as NRS (www.nrsweb.com) and Riversports (www.riversports.com), and check out the websites of raft, cataraft, and inflatable-kayak manufacturers, including Aire (www.aire.com), Jack's Plastic Welding (www.jpwinc.com), Hyside (www.hyside.com), and Star (www.starinflatables.com).

WATER TYPE

Obviously, it's best to start out on easier water and work your way up from there. Flatwater trips make fine river rafting experiences, particularly for toddlers who don't care much for rapids anyway. If, however, you're like most people and drawn to rafting for the opportunity to run rapids, you'll be able to start out safely with Class II and even some Class III water on your first do-it-yourself trip. (See page 218 for details on the whitewater rating system.)

On a guided trip, you and your kids can start out on up to Class IV water, with specific age limits set by outfitters (and their lawyers). On many guided river trips, outfitters provide inflatable kayaks to paddle—a terrific experience for youngsters and grown-ups alike.

If you're not overly experienced, you probably won't want to run Class IV water on your own with your kids on board until they're 9 or 10—old enough to take care of themselves and not panic should they be catapulted into the water while running a rapid. Unless you're tremendously experienced, you won't want them on board with you in Class V water until they're teenagers—at which point you may be better off with them at the oars than you.

Possibilities

NANTAHALA OUTDOOR CENTER

Nantahala Outdoor Center (NOC) has been guiding river trips (and providing whitewater paddling instruction) for more than 30 years from its base on the banks of the Nantahala River in western North Carolina.

The company offers half-day, full-day, and overnight trips on six area rivers: the Nantahala, Pigeon, Ocoee, French Broad, Nolichucky, and Chattooga.

NOC offers many trip variations. You'll have no difficulty choosing one that matches the age and adventurousness level of your kids, from the Class II and III water of the Nantahala River to the Class IV+ rapids of the Chattooga River, where the movie *Deliverance* was filmed. Possibilities include riding along with a guide/oarsperson, actively participating as a member of a paddle boat, captaining your own inflatable kayak, or renting your own raft for a do-it-your-self day trip.

Trips range in cost from $40 to $250 per person. For more information, call 888-905-7238 or visit www.noc.com.

ZOAR OUTDOOR

Zoar Outdoor provides kid-friendly day trips on three rivers that enable East Coast families to experience river rafting: the Millers and Deerfield rivers in Massachusetts and the West River in Vermont. The company is based in western Massachusetts, only two-and-a-half hours from Boston and three-and-a-half from New York City.

Zoar owner Karen Blom says most of the parents who sign their families up for the company's rafting trips are first-timers. "They may come back to do another trip or two with us, depending on the ages of their kids," says Blom. "Then a lot of them are ready for more."

At that point, Blom and her co-owner and husband, Bruce Leffels, offer their customers referrals to outfitters who run trips on other, more remote rivers in nearby Maine as well as in the Southeast and out West. "We're happy to give families their first taste of river running," says Blom, "and see many of them continue on from there."

Trips range in cost from $40 to $100 per person. For more information, call 800-532-7483 or visit www.zaroutdoor.com.

CANYON REO

Flagstaff, Arizona-based Canyon River Equipment Outfitters (REO) outfits do-it-yourselfers for trips on a number of rivers in the West. Though much of the company's business involves outfitting private Grand Canyon trips, Canyon REO provides gear and food for a number of rivers that are perfect for family outings, including the Chama River in New Mexico, the San Juan River in Utah, the Yampa River in Colorado, the Verde River in Arizona, the Salmon River in Idaho, and the Rogue River in Oregon.

In addition to outfitting do-it-yourself types, Canyon REO runs guided trips on a number of rivers in the Southwest through its sister company, Canyon Rio

Rafting. Three-quarters of the trips Canyon Rio runs include children, either as group members or as members of families.

Canyon REO/Rio owner Donnie Dove says the first time he ran a river with kids, he tried to run it the same as an adult trip. "I said, 'Okay, here we go. We're going to do 13 miles today, run this rapid and that rapid, and then make camp,'" Dove recalls.

He quickly learned that the idea of putting in lots of river miles, and lots of time seated in a raft, didn't work with kids. "I found out it's just as fun for adults—and a lot more fun for kids—to do the same 13 miles over two or even three days, to take time to skip rocks and search for mountain lions and play games," Dove says.

Canyon Rio tailors each trip for its participants. If parents want their kids to do some rock climbing as part of their family trip, for example, Canyon Rio guides are happy to oblige. If participants want lots of side-canyon hiking, no problem. If they lean toward lazing about on riverside beaches, that's fine, too.

Trips range in cost from $30 per person for a two-hour excursion to $825 per person for a five-day wilderness river adventure. For more information, call 800-272-3353 or visit www.canyonreo.com and/or www.canyonrio.com.

OARS

If Nantahala Outdoor Center is the granddaddy of southeastern river running, California-based Outdoor Adventure River Specialists (OARS) is the granddaddy of the West.

OARS was the first oar-powered outfitter permitted to run trips on the Colorado River through the Grand Canyon. That was back in 1969. Since then, OARS has grown to become the largest and most diverse river company in the West, running rivers in Idaho, Utah, California, Oregon, Wyoming, Alaska, and British Columbia.

Interested in running a river in the West with your kids, or, for that matter, one in some remote part of the world? It'll likely be on the OARS list.

Trips in the western US range in cost from $400 for a three-day trip on the Lower Klamath River in California to $5000 for a 21-day trip down the Grand Canyon. For more information, call 800-346-6277 or visit www.oars.com.

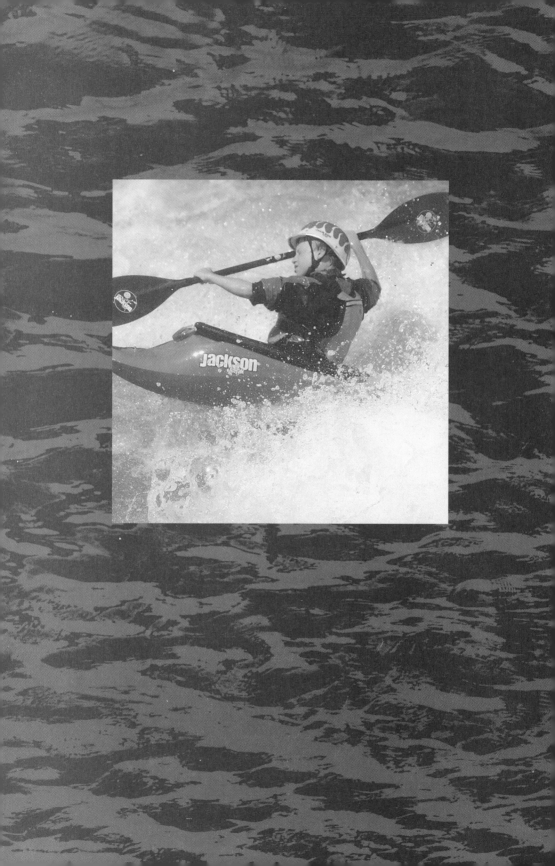

20 Whitewater Kayaking

Whitewater kayaking is booming. The Outdoor Industry Association reports there are nearly six million more kayakers in the US today than there were a few years ago, a 250 percent increase. Kayak sales are skyrocketing. Everybody, it seems, is taking up the sport—and with good reason. Whitewater kayaking is 100 percent, adrenaline-stoked fun.

I began looking forward to taking up hard-shell whitewater kayaking with my two boys shortly after they were born. Sue and I introduced kayaking to Taylor and Logan when each turned 6. These days, both are comfortable in their hard shells and are progressively becoming stronger and more capable paddlers.

As for me? I have yet to learn to roll—that is, to turn my hard shell back upright upon flipping upside down.

I'm the first to admit I'm not the most gifted of athletes. Still, I didn't imagine I'd have any trouble learning to roll a kayak, the single most critical kayaking skill.

Several parents I know who've set out to tackle kayaking with their kids find themselves where I am, struggling to master the roll while watching their kids learn the skill with ease. In one sense, I suppose, our struggles are emblematic of the lives we wish for our children. As parents, we want our children to achieve more than we have achieved, to go as far with their pursuits as their will, determination, and smarts will take them. But that sort of philosophizing doesn't make it easier to see your kids master a sport while you're still flailing.

If you already kayak and know how to roll, introducing kayaking to your kids will be relatively easy. You need simply get your kids geared up, take them out to some calm water—a swimming pool, lake, or flat stretch of river—and have at it.

It's parents who want to try out the sport for the first time along with their kids who may face some difficulty learning to roll a kayak, just as I have. Note, however, that you may just as well have little or no difficulty picking up the kayak roll.

"It's advanced weekend-warrior stuff as opposed to just weekend-warrior stuff," says former world-champion whitewater paddler Kent Ford of rolling a kayak back upright. "But the truth is, learning to roll isn't all that hard."

Through his Performance Video offerings and personal instruction, Ford has taught thousands of people to roll and kayak in whitewater. "There are lots of people out there in their 70s who have learned to roll," Ford says.

Hmm. Guess I'll keep trying.

> **The need for instruction is especially acute because of the safety issues involved with kayaking.**

Levels of Commitment

If you want to introduce your kids to whitewater kayaking and join them on the water yourself, you don't necessarily have to learn the roll. There are other opportunities for people at various levels of the sport:

Sticking with it until you master the roll. Kent Ford is, in fact, telling the truth when he says learning to roll a kayak isn't overly difficult. Perhaps you'll be one of those who master the roll right away. Perhaps it'll take you a while. Regardless, you'll need an instructor—either a friend or a paid teacher—to learn to roll a kayak successfully. Also, be sure to have a look at Ford's *The Kayak Roll*, widely regarded as the best kayak roll instructional video on the market (available at river sports stores and at www.performancevideo.com).

Settle for hard-shell kayaking without mastering a roll. Hard-shell kayakers who can't roll tend to take it easy when they're on the water. When they flip, they must exit from and swim to shore with their boats. They enjoy their downriver runs without turning upstream to surf holes because it's while surfing holes that most kayakers flip.

Go with an inflatable kayak. This is the route Sue and I have taken so far. We haven't yet given up on the idea of mastering the kayak roll. In the meantime, we run rivers in our mini-raft inflatable kayaks while Taylor and Logan run them in their hard shells.

Getting Your Kids Started

Given the various ways of taking on kayaking yourself, what's the best way to get your kids started?

When Sue and I were ready to introduce kayaking to Taylor at age 6, Performance Video's Kent Ford suggested simply throwing a boat in the water and throwing Taylor in with it. That approach works well as a way to get started. Very quickly, however, the need for instruction becomes crucial.

"A few days of lessons will reduce the chance of a bad experience," says Ford. "I've seen too many people get dragged too quickly into whitewater that wasn't conducive to learning, and then they end up quitting the sport." Three or four days of instruction provide the base all beginners need to progress as kayakers.

The need for instruction is especially acute because of the safety issues involved with kayaking. In terms of risk and danger, kayaking is similar to backcountry skiing: Just as backcountry skiers face the potential for avalanches and getting lost and disoriented in whiteout conditions, kayakers need to be careful about getting pinned against

The Basics

■ Kayaking lends itself well to families with children as young as 6.

■ Even if you don't learn the kayak roll, you still can join your kayaker kids on the water.

■ When it comes to taking on kayaking with your kids, sooner is better than later.

■ You can start your kids kayaking by throwing boats in the water and throwing your kids in with them. Very quickly, however, the need for instruction will become crucial.

rocks by rushing water. Both risks are associated with the ultimate power of nature.

Ford says kids, especially, need the grounding in precautionary measures provided by kayak instructors because learning to do things specifically with safety in mind doesn't come naturally to children.

"Kids are going to learn the 'sport' part of kayaking faster than they're going to learn kayaking's safety protocols," Ford says. "They're not accustomed to learning that sort of safety information—and parents must keep that in mind."

In response to the growing demand, many whitewater instruction centers are now offering clinics for entire families. Some of those centers are listed in the Possibilities section at the end of this chapter (page 230). You can locate others, possibly closer to your home, by searching the internet and checking in with your local river sports store.

Paddler magazine has an extensive list of whitewater kayak schools on its website, www.paddlermagazine.com (keyword: Tripfinder). *WaveLength* magazine also has a list of kayak schools on its website, www.wavelength-magazine.com. Both magazines' sites provide good introductory reading about the sport of kayaking.

Age Limits

When it comes to taking on kayaking with your kids, sooner is better than later. It's far better to instill caution and good judgment in your kids when they're youngsters and you're on the water with them than have them learn the sport with their buddies as teenagers, when safety will be far down on their list of priorities.

Many kayaking schools don't accept children under age 10, but some, such as Four Corners Riversports in Durango, are allowing kids as young as 6 as more parents turn their youngsters on to the sport.

Riversports co-owner Andy Corra says when Riversports first started kids' classes, the school's age minimum was 10. Then came the introduction of kayaking equipment suitable for younger children. "We started a class for 8- and 9-year-olds," says Corra, "but we had parents calling us up asking about classes for kids as young as 5. We decided 5 was too young, but we now have a Tadpole class for 6- and 7-year-olds."

Corra says the Tadpole class has proven popular, even though instruction takes place in a pool and on a local lake, as opposed to on flowing water.

These days, 60 percent of Four Corners Riversports' kayak students are kids. "And the flip side," says Corra, "is that the kids taking our courses are turning around and pulling their parents into the sport."

Corra attributes much of the youth-kayaking boom to the "park-and-play phenomenon." Many of the kayaks sold today are playboats, which means they're designed not for river running, but for staying in one place and surfing the same hole over and over. As a result, parents and kids can play in one place on a river for an hour or two at a time, with no car shuttles required.

Assuming you want to join your kids on the water rather than just watch them from shore, park-and-play kayaking will work for you as a parent only if you know

When it comes to taking on kayaking with your kids, sooner is better than later.

Kayak Gear for Kids

Let's be honest: Kayaking is gear intensive. Even buying used where possible, you're looking at several hundred dollars to outfit each of your kids for the sport. The best way to try out the sport is by renting. Rental outfits typically provide all the gear, including boat, spray skirt, paddle, helmet, PFD, and clothing.

In 2004, when Rock Island, Tennessee-based Jackson Kayak (www.jacksonkayak.com) introduced the miniature Fun 1 **boat** for kid paddlers weighing up to 80 pounds, whitewater kayaking became possible for small children.

Until the Fun 1, several boat models were marketed to children, particularly the Jib by Perception (www.kayaker.com), the Evo by Wavesport (www.wavesport.com), and the Blast by Dagger (www.dagger.com). Those three boats are now discontinued, but they are still available on the used market. Taylor and Logan paddle a Jib and a Blast. While these boats are acceptable for juniors, they aren't easy for kids to handle because they're significantly larger than the Fun 1—large enough, in fact, to accommodate small adults.

Unfortunately, the Fun 1 and another in the series, the Fun 1.5, which is good for kids who weigh 100 pounds, are not yet widely available on the used market. The Fun 1 retails for $700 and the Fun 1.5 sells for $800.

A less expensive way to start your kids kayaking is

to pick up used Jibs, Evos, Blasts, or other boats designed for small adults for $150 or $200 each online. (You'll get almost the same amount of money for the boats when you resell them later.)

Jackson recently introduced a line of short kayak **paddles** to go with its kid-size boats. The paddles are available as short as 150 centimeters, though kids can get away with using short adult paddles (in the 190-centimeter range).

Lotus Designs (www.lotusdesigns.com) makes the Half-Pint **PFD** for kids up to 90 pounds. Kids who weigh more than 90 pounds can use PFDs for small adults.

Grateful Heads (www.gratefulheads.com) makes the Edge **helmet**, which comes in an extra-extra small size for small heads. Shred Ready (www.shredready.com) makes the Vixen for small women's (and kids') heads. The Vixen comes in acceptable colors for boys; just don't mention that the helmet is meant for women.

If your kids will be paddling in cool or cold water, a **drytop** will be an essential piece of equipment. A drytop is a water-proof pullover jacket with rubber gaskets at the wrists and neck to keep the wearer entirely dry and, as a result, warm. Lotus Designs makes its River Rotator drytop in an extra-small size, with neck and wrist gaskets tight enough to fit children.

A number of extra-small **spray skirts** will work for kids. When they're very young, your kids can kayak without spray skirts. As they get older, they'll need spray skirts in order to keep their boats from filling with water when they lean back and forth, even before they learn to roll. In addition to spray skirts, any number of small-size neoprene shorts and any assortment of kid-size polypropylene tops and bottoms, as necessary for warmth, will work for kids.

Finally, correctly sized specialty whitewater **earplugs** are essential to protect the ear canals of your young kayakers if they get into the sport to the point where they're rolling a great deal, especially in cold water.

how—or can learn—to roll a kayak. Conversely, you'll find downriver kayaking a great sport to enjoy with your kids even if, like me, you don't manage to master the kayak roll right away.

Possibilities

ZOAR OUTDOOR

Charlemont, Massachusetts-based Zoar Outdoor provides a great opportunity for members of families in the Northeast to try the sport of kayaking together. For several years, Zoar Outdoor, located on the banks of the Deerfield River in western Massachusetts, has offered two-day parent/child novice whitewater kayaking clinics. In 2004, Zoar began offering its Family Kayak Week, a full week of kayaking instruction designed to take an entire family from novice to intermediate in a few intense days.

Each June, Zoar holds its DemoFest weekend, during which participants can try out a variety of the latest kayak models, including the Jackson Fun 1 and 1.5.

Zoar's two-day parent/child novice kayaking clinic costs $265 for adults and $240 for children. The Family Kayak Week costs $495 for adults and $395 for children. For more information, call 800-532-7483 or go to www.zaaroutdoor.com.

> You'll find downriver kayaking a great sport to enjoy with your kids, even if you don't manage to master the kayak roll right away.

NANTAHALA OUTDOOR CENTER

Unlike Zoar Outdoor, Bryson City, North Carolina-based Nantahala Outdoor Center (NOC), the largest whitewater instruction school in the country, does not offer a specific kayak instruction course for families. Instead, at its base on the banks of the Nantahala River in western North Carolina, NOC offers private group instruction packages for parents and children who want to learn to kayak together.

"One of the things families need is more time together," says Wayne Dickert, NOC's instruction manager. "Our private instruction courses for families give them that opportunity."

After taking an introductory private family course from NOC, many families split up to take courses at various levels, Dickert says. He reports that kid kayak instruction is the fastest growing portion of NOC's whitewater instruction program.

A day of private instruction for a family of four, including lunch and all equipment, runs $500. For more information, call 888-905-7238 or go to www.noc.com.

SUNDANCE RIVER CENTER

Merlin, Oregon-based Sundance River Center offers family kayak instruction programs from its base on the banks of the Rogue River in southwestern Oregon.

The outfitter's Family Kayak School teaches parents and children who want to learn to kayak together. Children receive a 10 percent discount when they enroll in any of the center's classes at the same time as their parents.

For more information, call 888-777-7557 or go to www.sundanceriver.com.

CANYON RIO

If you and your kids have tried hard-shell kayaking and want more instruction, consider working your way up the learning curve by joining a Canyon Rio kayak instruction river trip.

Rather than teach kayak skills to families in one

place
like most kayak
instruction schools, Flagstaff,
Arizona-based Canyon Rio combines kayak instruction
with three-day trips each summer down either the San
Juan River in Utah or the Chama River in New Mexico.

Canyon Rio's unique river trip/instruction course offers
you and your kids the best of both worlds: a fun wilderness river journey, plus kayak instruction along the way.
Canyon Rio accepts paddlers as young as 7 on its kayak-
instruction trips, provided they have appropriate previous
experience. The three-day trips cost $475 per person.

For more information, call 800-272-3353 or go to
www.canyonrio.com.

HIT THE ROAD

Once you and your kids have mastered basic kayaking
techniques, the nation's rivers can be your playground.
You may even be inspired to follow in the paddle strokes
of the Jackson family: pro-kayaker dad Eric, mom Kristine,
US Junior Freestyle Team member and daughter Emily,
and US Junior Freestyle Team member and son Dane.
Since Emily and Dane were youngsters, the Jacksons have
spent about 200 days a year kayaking.

Even if you don't quit your job and imitate the Jacksons
after you take up the sport, a week or two of road-trip

kayaking can make for a terrific family vacation. One idea for such a trip would be to visit one or more of the growing number of whitewater parks being constructed in urban settings on rivers around the country. The Susquehanna Whitewater Park Alliance maintains an online list of these parks in the US and Europe. Go to www.swwparkalliance.com (keywords: Whitewater Parks Around the Globe).

For more of a backcountry experience, try working off the list of 150 US rivers officially designated as Wild and Scenic by the federal government. Visit www.nps.gov/rivers (keywords: Designated WSRs) for the list and information on those rivers.

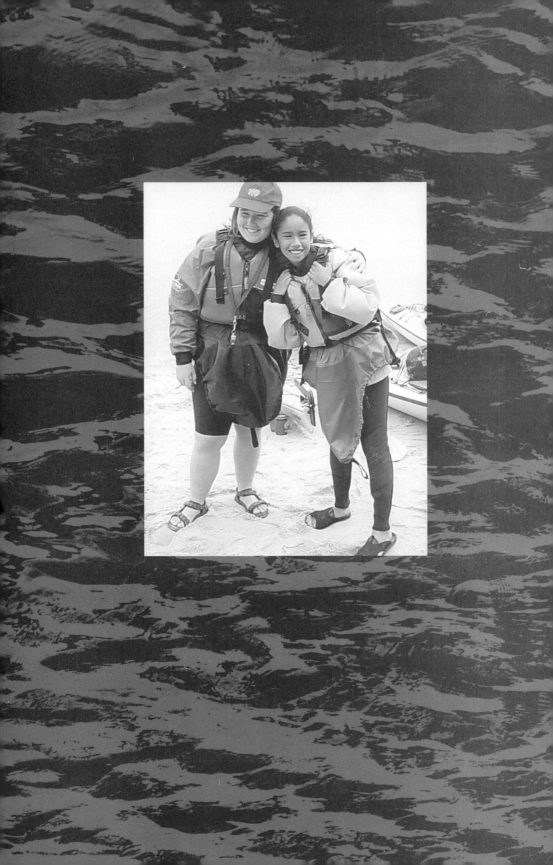

21 Flatwater Canoeing and Sea Kayaking

I t's true that rapids put much of the "extreme" in backcountry trips involving water travel, but there's still great fun to be had canoeing and kayaking lakes, calm rivers, and ocean waters with kids.

Over the last few years, my family has run most of the exciting whitewater rivers within driving distance of our home, but one of the best family river trips we've taken was on the flatwater stretch of Utah's Green River through Labyrinth Canyon. The broad, slow-flowing Green carried us along the same route taken by Major John Wesley Powell and his men, who boated the Green River to its confluence with the Colorado River and on through the Grand Canyon in 1869. We didn't run any rapids, but we had a terrific time jumping from our boats, floating along in the river in our PFDs, playing on the beaches along the way, and exploring desert side canyon after desert side canyon.

Labyrinth Canyon, with its stunning ocher and red sandstone walls, is just one of countless flatwater river and lake journeys awaiting you and your kids virtually everywhere in the country.

By Canoe

As family backcountry trips go, it's hard to beat taking off into the wilderness by canoe with your kids. Together, you can explore a remote lake, series of lakes, or flatwater stretch of river. Like river rafting trips and llama-supported backpacking trips, flatwater canoe trips enable you and your kids to get away from cars and roads without hauling everything you need on your backs.

There are many great reasons to go by canoe:

Backcountry canoe trips are simple. Renting canoes and associated gear is cheap and easy. Rental canoes and gear are widely available near popular flatwater-trip locations for $50 to $100 a day. Beyond that, you need nothing more than car-camping supplies—though outfitters even provide camping gear and food for more popular trips such as those into Minnesota's Boundary Waters Canoe Area Wilderness. You need only some car-camping experience to pull off a simple, warm-weather canoe trip not far from civilization with your kids. From there, you can gradually up the arduousness of your trips to the extent you wish.

The Basics

- There's great fun to be had canoeing and kayaking lakes, calm rivers, and ocean waters with kids.

- Renting canoes and associated gear is cheap and easy.

- Tremendous flatwater canoe trips on quiet lakes and calm rivers exist in most parts of the country.

- In addition to providing the means to paddle ocean and large lake waters, a pair of two-person sea kayaks provides an excellent method of conveyance for two parents and two kids taking inland trips on smaller lakes and flatwater rivers where canoes might normally be used.

They're exciting in a relatively safe way. On a backcountry flatwater trip, you will enjoy the same awe and wonder of going off into the middle of nowhere as you would on a whitewater river trip, but without the trepidation and required whitewater-paddling skills and/or hired guides that are part of any river trip involving rapids.

They're everywhere. Tremendous flatwater canoe trips on quiet lakes and calm rivers exist in most parts of the country. Such trips number, literally, in the thousands. For a state-by-state list of outfitters and potential trips, go to www.americaoutdoors.org.

They don't demand a whole lot of advance planning. While the possibilities for private-party backcountry whitewater trips are limited in the US (the best whitewater trips

Canoes vs. Sea Kayaks

Because of their closed cockpits, sea kayaks can be used on any flatwater trip. Open canoes, on the other hand, are susceptible to swamping by high waves, and so are used only where high waves aren't an issue.

The closed cockpits of sea kayaks make them more problematic than canoes for hauling gear because everything carried on a sea kayak trip must fit through the kayaks' small hatches.

often involve applying for and winning permits in lotteries months in advance), most flatwater trips do not involve the same crush of people. The result? You can decide Friday afternoon to spend your weekend canoeing, and be at a quiet put-in, ready to go, Saturday morning.

By Sea Kayak

The complexities of weather, large waves, and large-boat traffic make taking to the ocean or large lakes with children in sea kayaks more demanding than inland flatwater trips on rivers or smaller lakes by canoe or sea kayak. Still, family trips by sea kayak on the ocean or large lakes are entirely doable. You can tackle a guided sea kayak trip with no previous experience. If you're a do-it-yourselfer, however, you'll most likely want to begin by going out with your kids in sea kayaks for a day trip or two before trying an overnight adventure.

In addition to providing the means to paddle ocean waters, a pair of two-person sea kayaks provides an excellent method of conveyance for two parents and two kids taking inland trips on lakes and flatwater rivers where canoes might normally be used.

Annual Trip

Many families with kids swear by the annual backcountry flatwater trips they take together. Every summer, the six members of the Mummery family—dad John, mom Mary, and four kids—explore by canoe a different section of northern Minnesota's Boundary Waters Canoe Area

Wilderness, the ultimate flatwater canoe trip destination in the country.

John says a Boundary Waters trip is the perfect backcountry family getaway. "Plus, our Boundary Waters trips are easy to pull off," he says, "which, with four kids, is an important factor."

The Mummerys rent boats and gear from an outfitter when they arrive at the Boundary Waters. "Our trips are affordable," John continues. "Canoeing the Boundary Waters is something we can do in the backcountry with our kids that doesn't require us to hire guides or be part of an expensive outfitted expedition. Instead, we just pay the $50 or so a day to rent each of our boats, and that's it."

John recommends renting lightweight Kevlar canoes, even though rates for such canoes generally are higher than for heavier canoes. "With lightweight canoes, you can really get a long ways into the backcountry," John says. "They make any portages you have to do incredibly easy."

If you're planning an annual trip with your family, follow these hints for an easy and enjoyable flatwater trip with your kids:

Hire help. Don't be afraid to hire a guide, either for a few hours to give you pointers, or to accompany you on your entire first flatwater canoe or sea kayak trip.

Even though paddling flatwater requires less skill than whitewater, there's a great deal of knowledge to be gained from an expert, and that knowledge is worth its minimal cost because it will serve you well in subsequent trips.

> The shorter and simpler the first flatwater paddling trips you tackle with your kids, the happier you and they will be.

Take advantage of technology. John and Mary Mummery take a GPS unit and a fish finder on their paddle-and-portage Boundary Waters canoe trips with their kids.

The GPS unit provides peace of mind when John and Mary venture deep into the backcountry and each lake they paddle begins to look like the last.

The fish finder has a more important purpose: to measure water depth below lakeside cliffs near potential campsites. "We always try to camp near shoreline cliffs that have adequate water depth beneath them," says John. "The kids spend lots of their camp time jumping from the cliffs into the water, which gives Mary and me a chance to relax."

Other technological advances are worth the investment as well. For example, lightweight camping gear makes portages easier, and the lighter weight of Kevlar canoes makes them worth their higher rental fees.

Start small. Starting small, a theme of this book, certainly applies here.

It may seem that flatwater paddling is fairly simple: You just get in the boat and go. The reality, however, is that there are many skills you'll pick up only after several flatwater trips. You'll use more energy packing, paddling, choosing campsites, loading and unloading gear from your boats, and setting up and taking down camps on your first trips than you will on subsequent trips. That means the shorter and simpler the first trips you tackle with your kids, the happier you and they will be.

Go light. If you'll be doing a paddle-and-portage trip, weight will be a particular concern. Even on flatwater river trips that don't involve portaging, weight can become an issue.

The gear-hauling capability of canoes and sea kayaks means you can take a lot of gear with you on non-portage flatwater trips into the backcountry—but you will have to load and unload whatever you take along at every campsite.

Camp tables and chairs, gas lanterns, two-burner stoves, large tents, coolers filled with ice and beer—all are nice to have in camp. But are they worth loading and unloading day after day? You'll have to be the judge.

Possibilities

BOUNDARY WATERS CANOE AREA WILDERNESS

Paddling Minnesota's one-million-acre Boundary Waters Canoe Area Wilderness is considered by many the premier flatwater canoe trip in the country. People come from around the world to paddle the wilderness area's 1200 miles of canoe routes across hundreds of lakes and connecting rivers in far northern Minnesota's Superior National Forest.

> **Paddling the Boundary Waters is considered by many the premier flatwater canoe trip in the country.**

Numerous outfitters in and around the town of Ely, Minnesota, serve the more than 200,000 people who visit the Boundary Waters wilderness each year. Most outfitters provide whatever level of outfitting customers want—from a shuttle ride to a put-in point to complete packages that include canoes, all camping gear, and food. Most outfitters also help customers select a trip and route and obtain a permit.

"The number of lakes and route possibilities is limitless, so we help map out each trip for our customers as they make their plans," explains Dave Sebesta, manager of Williams and Hall Wilderness Guides and Outfitters (800-322-5837; www.williamsandhall.com) in Ely. "We get details from the family or group members—their interests, the amount of time they have, their physical abilities, what they're trying to get out of their trip—and we custom-tailor each trip from there."

Sebesta estimates that more than a third of Williams and Hall's business is serving families, while another third of the outfitter's business is made up of youth groups such

as
Scout troops.
The fact that more than
two-thirds of the outfitter's business involves children makes sense, says
Sebesta: With all its swimming, fishing, and easy-and-fun-
paddling possibilities, the Boundary Waters wilderness is
perfect for kids.

The primary Boundary Waters season runs from May
through September; mid-July to mid-August is the busiest
time period. Mosquito numbers in any given location vary
widely from year to year, and even from month to month
and week to week.

The first six to eight hours from any Boundary Waters
entry point tend to be heavily traveled during the summer
months. Those who paddle and portage away from an
entry point for more than a day, however, will see a dra-
matic decrease in the number of people, even during the
height of the summer season.

To learn more about the Boundary Waters permit and
quota system, visit www.bwcaw.org. Serious about a
Boundary Waters trip? Check out the Wilderness Press
Boundary Waters Canoe Area guides, volumes one and two,
by Robert Beymer. The incredibly detailed maps published
by Fisher Maps (www.fishermaps.com) are the mainstay
of Boundary Waters canoeists.

LABYRINTH AND STILLWATER CANYONS

While the Boundary Waters is the top place for a flatwater wilderness lake trip in the country, the 120-mile
stretch of Utah's Green River through Labyrinth and
Stillwater canyons is considered by many the premier flatwater wilderness river trip in the US.

Sue and I canoed Labyrinth and Stillwater canyons, from
the town of Green River, Utah, to the Green's confluence

with the Colorado River in the heart of Canyonlands National Park, before the boys were born. The trip was so phenomenal—and seemed so great for kids—that we returned to repeat it, with great success, when the boys were toddlers.

The Labyrinth-Stillwater stretch of the Green is primarily wilderness, with limited road access points. You and your kids can paddle just Labyrinth Canyon, just

Stillwater Canyon, or both canyons. You'll need five or six days to float either canyon, or 10 to 12 days to float both (more if you factor in layover days for long side-canyon hikes and beach play).

Tex's Riverway Adventures (435-259-5101; www.texsriverways.com) is the primary outfitter supplying shuttles plus canoe and gear rental services for Labyrinth and Stillwater trips. From its base in Moab, Utah, the outfitter operates bus shuttles to three put-in/take-out points along the Labyrinth/Stillwater stretch of the Green. In addition, the company operates a jet boat that runs down the Colorado River from Moab to pick up paddlers who float the Green through Stillwater Canyon to the confluence of the Green and Colorado rivers.

(Your kids may well declare the noisy ride back up the Colorado to Moab on the jet boat the highlight of their

Green River float trip. Don't be fooled, however. They'll have loved the trip itself, with its sandy beaches and nights beneath the stars.)

A Labyrinth/Stillwater trip is similar to any flatwater river trip in that watercraft skills and paddling knowledge are secondary to camping and wilderness- and desert-travel know-how. The Green River will carry you downstream to where you want to go (though high winds can be a serious factor). More important will be your and your kids' ability to safely and enjoyably take on bugs, mud, sun, silt, cactus, and sharp rocks.

SAN JUAN ISLANDS

Like green emeralds rising from the waters of Washington's Puget Sound, the San Juan Islands northwest of Seattle arguably comprise the nation's most picturesque sea kayaking destinations. They're certainly the most popular.

Vacationers flock to the San Juans from July through September, when the sun shines consistently over the islands. Many visitors sea kayak as part of their visits; most rent boats for day trips. Several outfitters offer visitors multiday camping trips among the islands. Discovery Sea Kayaks (360-378-2559; www.discoverysea-kayaks.com), for example, offers multiday family trips complete with three-seat kayaks so that small children may travel safely between two paddling adults. Older children take the fore seat in Discovery's two-seater boats and help with the paddling. Discovery limits the group size of its multiday trips to six. The outfitter's three- and five-day trips cost about $150 per person per day.

In addition to full-service expeditions, Discovery offers trips that include only rental boats and a guide, enabling you to save money by bringing your own food and

> **The San Juan Islands arguably comprise the nation's most picturesque sea kayaking destination.**

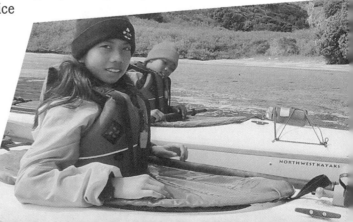

camping gear. These self-catered trips cost about $90 per person per day.

Many families with sea kayaking experience undertake San Juan trips on their own. If you're considering a do-it-yourself San Juan sea kayak trip, be sure to check out *Kayaking Puget Sound, the San Juans, and Gulf Islands*, by Randel Washburne and R. Carey Gersten (Mountaineers Books, 1999).

CASCO BAY ISLANDS

On the East Coast, only 100 miles from Boston, the Maine Island Kayak Company offers a pair of three-day family sea kayak trips from the outfitter's headquarters near Portland, Maine, on Peaks Island in Casco Bay.

The company's trip for families with children ages 10 to 12 is more for the experience of paddling a sea kayak than for putting in lots of miles. During the trip, families use double-cockpit kayaks to explore islands in southern Casco Bay, near the company's headquarters. Highlights of the trip include the exploration of tidal pools, pocket beaches, lighthouses, and abandoned forts.

The outfitter's longer-mileage trip for families with children ages 13 to 16 offers older kids the opportunity to paddle their own, single-cockpit boats.

Maine Island Kayak Company's three-day family trips run about $400 per person. For more information, call 800-796-2373 or go to www.maineislandkayak.com.

APOSTLE ISLANDS NATIONAL LAKESHORE

A trip to the Apostle Islands off the northern Wisconsin coast in Lake Superior ranks high in the family sea kayaking adventurousness scale.

The cold waters of Lake Superior, prone to fog, storms, and high waves, are suitable only for experienced sea kayaking families. Wetsuits or drysuits are essential equipment for a trip to the Apostles, where the risk of hypothermia is high. In addition, paddlers must pack additional provisions because regular weather delays prevent movement from island to island and back to the mainland.

All that said, the federally protected Apostle Islands offer tremendous sea kayaking opportunities to the stout of heart. See www.nps.gov/apis to learn more.

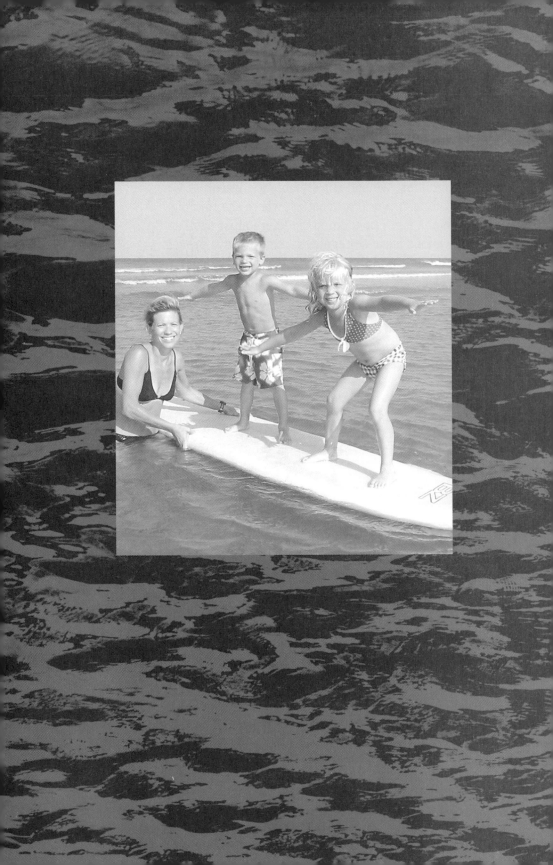

22 Bodyboarding and Surfing

The sports of surfing and bodyboarding offer kids and adults alike the potential for endless outdoor fun. Unlike many other outdoor sports that are more gear intensive, these two surf sports are relatively inexpensive. Your biggest expense, in fact, won't be the gear you'll have to rent or buy in order to try out either sport with your kids. Rather, assuming you don't live near a beach with rideable waves, your biggest expense will be getting to one.

When it comes to surfing in particular, a second expense—but a worthwhile one, according to parents who have introduced their kids to the sport—is a lesson. Dana Siekman signed her three children up for a day of lessons on the North Carolina coast when they were 8, 9, and 10.

"It was perfect," says Siekman. "The surf was rough that day, but the instructors were expert at making the kids feel okay in the choppy water." Moreover, says Siekman, the instructors looked the part of surfer dudes, something her children relished.

"The instructors got the kids in the water quickly and got going with them," says Siekman. "By the end of one lesson, my kids knew how to surf. It was awesome."

Vicki Whiting introduced surfing to her oldest son, Phillip, during a West Coast vacation when he turned 12. She was amazed at how quickly Phillip—like the Siekman kids—picked up the sport. "Fifteen, 20 minutes, that's all it took," Whiting says. "After that, he was standing on the board, riding. And he loved every minute of it."

Bodyboarding rivals surfing on the fun scale, and it's even easier for youngsters to learn.

As with scuba diving and kiteboarding (the final two outdoor sports covered in this book), bodyboarding and surfing aren't backcountry sports—but they're truly fun, truly extreme, and truly family friendly.

Bodyboarding

Bodyboarding (or boogie boarding)—riding ocean waves on short, squat, foam-core boards—is a particularly simple sport to pick up. In fact, its simplest form is so easy to learn and perform that surfers are known to disparage the sport and call bodyboarders "spongers" for taking up space in wave trains that many surfers believe ought to be theirs.

The reality, however, is that bodyboarding, like surfing, is a legitimate sport that even has its own governing body, the International Bodyboarding Association, and a professional tour (www.iba-tour.com). The extreme aspect of bodyboarding—riding monster waves à la upright surfers—has boomed internationally in recent years, and the bodyboarding industry is working to bring that boom to the US. In the meantime, bodyboarding remains to most

Americans a recreational pastime. In that form, bodyboarding is a fantastic sport to take on with your youngsters when they're as young as 4.

Sue and I brought a pair of inexpensive bodyboards along on a recent trip we took with Taylor and Logan to Costa Rica. We'd planned to do all the things families are supposed to do during visits to that country— see the mountainous cloud forest, hike to remote waterfalls deep in the lowland rain forest, and visit butterfly farms and wildlife preserves. Instead, when the boys discovered how much fun it was to ride Costa Rica's manageable waves on the boards we'd brought along, bodyboarding became the primary focus of our vacation.

The Basics

■ Unlike many other outdoor sports that are more gear intensive, bodyboarding and surfing are relatively inexpensive.

■ An introductory surf lesson for your kids is a worthwhile expense.

■ Bodyboarding rivals surfing on the fun scale, and it's even easier for youngsters to learn.

■ Surf schools dot both US coasts. Florida's relatively warm water temperatures and generally low and regular waves make its camps top destinations for beginners. Still, most US surf is gentle enough for learning purposes.

We wound up spending much of our trip working our way up and down Costa Rica's Pacific Coast, searching for secluded beaches with waves suitable for bodyboarding. The search was fun: We followed steep trails down to hidden coves and hiked long spits of sand, all in search of decent surf. The boarding was even better. Our only regret was that we brought along only two boards, which meant two members of the family had to wait impatiently while the other two members boarded.

Bodyboarding in waves up to 2 feet high is simple and safe enough for youngsters to try. They need simply walk into the surf, turn their backs to the waves, tuck their boards against their bellies, and ride a breaking wave to shore.

Obviously, the larger the wave, the more fun the ride. But larger waves require more finesse to catch—and they can pummel the unwary.

Advanced bodyboarding is a truly extreme sport. Top bodyboarders use fins to propel themselves down the faces of huge waves, the appearance of which, generally

Surf Lingo

More than perhaps any other extreme outdoor sport, surfing uses its own terminology. Here's a short, beginner-oriented glossary:

Angling: Surfing across the face of a wave at an angle rather than surfing a wave straight in toward shore. When your kids begin angling, they'll have moved beyond the realm of pure beginner.

Bomb: An unusually large wave in a set.

Carving: When a talented surfer carves up the face of a wave using his surfboard like a knife.

Deck: Top surface of a surfboard.

Face: The shoreward front of a wave, where most surfing takes place.

Goofyfoot: Surfer who surfs right-foot forward.

Grom or Grommet: A young surfer.

Kook: Surfer who thinks he's better than he really is. Often applied to beginners.

Lineup: Area of the ocean where surfers wait to catch waves.

Longboard: A surfboard that is longer, broader, and more buoyant than a conventional, shorter board. Recommended for beginners.

Pop-up: The move from lying to standing upright on a surfboard.

Rail: Edge of a surfboard.

Rubber Arms: The feeling of weakened arm muscles after lots of paddling. Often felt by beginners.

Set: A series of waves approaching the lineup.

Shredding: Advanced carving.

Soft board: Beginner surfboard with a soft deck.

Waterman: A person who boasts all oceanic skills—ability to surf, kiteboard, dive, spearfish, save drowning persons, etc., all in a single bound. Perhaps your kids will be watermen someday.

associated with storm systems, they (and surfers) track religiously at websites such as www.surfline.com and www.surfinfo.com.

Surfing

Surfing is best introduced to kids ages 8 and up. While basic bodyboarding generally is a do-it-yourself endeavor (though bodyboarding instruction is available), basic surfing instruction is a good idea.

Surf schools dot both US coasts. East Coast hot spots include Florida, North Carolina, and Long Island, New York. On the West Coast, many surf schools call the southern coast of California home. A smattering of schools service the cooler waters of northern California, while camps are rare in the cold waters of coastal Oregon and Washington. From among the dozens of surf schools, the possibilities listed at the end of this chapter are those that include something extra for families beyond the normal surf-school experience.

Florida's relatively warm water temperatures and generally low and regular waves make its camps top destinations for beginners. Still, most US surf is gentle enough for learning purposes. The best bet for finding a surf camp where you want to go? Surf the internet.

If you and your kids grow proficient at surfing, you'll be ready to take on bigger waves around the world. Hawaii is a top destination for upper-level surfers, as is Costa Rica.

251

(Hawaii's crowded Waikiki Beach is a popular beginner surf beach as well.)

To steep yourself in the surfing world (and to accomplish the all-important step of learning a handful of surfing terms so you'll sound cool to your kids) visit www.surfingthemag.com and www.surfermag.com. In addition, the Surfology section of www.surfline.com offers lots of good advice for beginning surfers.

Possibilities

COROLLA SURF SCHOOL

At the far north end of North Carolina's Outer Banks islands sits the village of Corolla and the Corolla Surf School.

Though vacation mansions and shopping plazas are sprouting up in the area, Corolla remains about as far off the beaten path as it's possible to get on the East Coast. Despite, or perhaps because of, Corolla's out-of-the-way status, the Corolla Surf School receives high marks from its customers.

Surf and Bodyboard Gear for Kids

The inexpensive Styrofoam **bodyboards** sold at sporting-goods stores wear out after a few days of use. If you and your kids plan to do some serious bodyboarding, you'll want to invest in higher-end boards, which run $80 to $200.

Because of riptide concerns, both Taylor and Logan wore **PFDs** while boarding in Costa Rica. If a rip had taken them out to sea—not an uncommon occurrence along Costa Rica's Pacific Coast—their PFDs would have kept them afloat. Depending on the age and swimming abilities of your children and the locations you'll be engaging in surf play with them, requiring your kids to use PFDs may be worth considering.

Bigger surf and fewer crowds await you along the Oregon and Washington coasts, but you'll need **wetsuits** to brave those chillier waters. Conversely, in sunnier climes, long-sleeved rash-guard shirts are worthwhile attire—and will make your kids feel like true members of the surfer crowd.

Surfboards cost $200 to $400. It's probably worth renting first to see if your kids like the sport. If you do buy, be sure your kids demo—try out the different boards you are considering—before you make a purchase.

Your kids' first boards should have plenty of volume; that is, they should be long and thick for lots of buoyancy. The short, skinnier, dagger-shaped boards of surfer-flick fame are for big waves and experts only.

Most families rent vacation homes by the week when they visit Corolla. In general, Corolla is less expensive than busier towns farther south on North Carolina's Outer Banks.

The Corolla Surf School offers bodyboarding as well as surfing lessons. Because its classes fill early during the busy summer months, the school suggests making reservations for instruction as far in advance as possible. A two-hour introductory lesson for families with kids ages 9 and up costs $60 per person.

For more information, call 252-453-9283 or visit www.corolla-surfshop.com. For more about visiting Corolla, go to www.outer-banks.com/corolla.

WRIGHTSVILLE BEACH SURF CAMP

You'll face more crowds at the southern end of North Carolina's coast than you will at the northern end, but you'll enjoy the camaraderie of other families if you sign up for Wrightsville Beach Surf Camp's Family Surf Camp Week, offered each summer to families with children ages 8 and up.

The school's family week features days of surf instruction on any or all of four developed barrier islands, depending on surf conditions. Those days are interspersed with visits to the North Carolina Aquarium, a nearby sea-turtle hospital, and an undeveloped barrier island.

Wrightsville Beach Surf Camp bills itself as an ecological outfitter with instructors schooled in marine science as well as surf instruction.

Wrightsville Beach is considered by *Surfing* magazine as one of the top 10 surf beaches in the country. Learning to surf at Wrightsville Beach will put you in the middle of the surfing world, something your kids will love.

The family surf camp is $295 per person for five days, with two or three hours of lessons per day. For more information about Wrightsville Beach Surf Camp, call 866-844-7873 or visit www.wbsurfcamp.com.

Learning to surf at Wrightsville Beach will put you in the middle of the surfing world, something your kids will love.

DO-IT-YOURSELF BODYBOARDING AND SURFING

This book is focused primarily on outdoor action sports in the US, but if you're interested in getting away from the crowds for some bodyboarding or surfing in warm water, you'll be hard pressed to do so within the country's borders.

Costa Rica's many quiet beaches, particularly those on the Nicoya Peninsula and south of Manuel Antonio National Park on the country's Pacific Coast, lend themselves well to such adventurousness with kids, though getting yourself and your kids to the country isn't cheap.

For a less expensive alternative, consider working your way south along Mexico's Baja Peninsula from San Diego for a week or two of beach and wave play without the California crowds.

Visit www.wannasurf.com and www.globalsurfers.com for up-to-the-minute descriptions of surf spots and breaks around the world. Also check out *The Stormrider Guide: North America* and *The World Stormrider Guide* for profiles by expert surfers of the best surf spots on the planet. (*Stormrider* guides are distributed by Wilderness Press.)

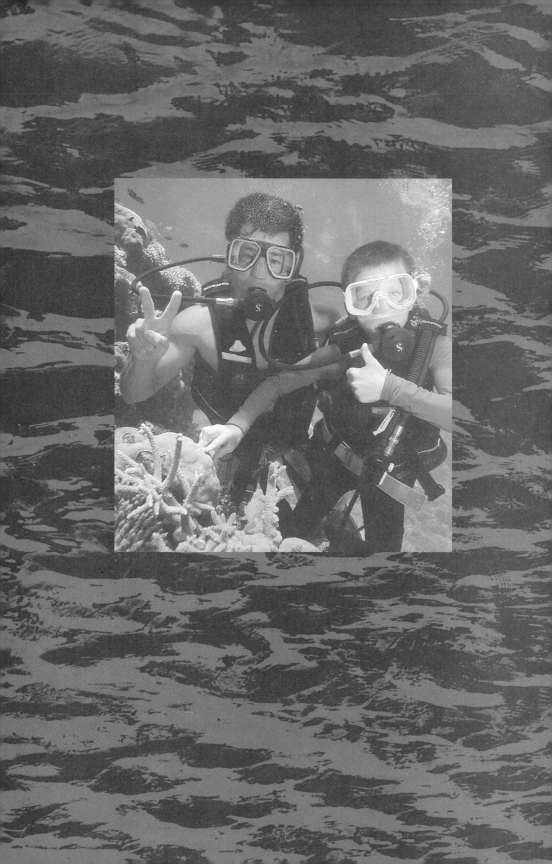

23 Scuba Diving

S cuba diving is another of those sports that can vex adults—all that bulky equipment, trying to get the hang of breathing underwater, figuring out how to use a regulator—while many kids pick it up quickly.

John Mummery remembers the first scuba course taken by his son, Colin. The class consisted of teenagers, adults, and Colin, then 10. John sat at the side of the pool watching.

"The instructor had all the class members lined up in the shallow end, working with their equipment," Mummery recalls. "He was showing them how to use their regulators, how to breathe, all the things you have to figure out before you can dive."

John's attention wandered. When he glanced back at the class, it took him a moment to locate Colin.

The instructor was still explaining everything to all the members of the class—except Colin, who by then was lying nonchalantly on his back at the bottom of the pool, breathing through his regulator and looking up at the rest of the class members while waiting for them to join him underwater.

As it is for so many outdoor sports, so it is with diving: Want to try the sport with your kids? Go right ahead, and be prepared for you, not them, to be the laggard on the learning curve.

Certification

The first step you and your kids must take to explore the sport of scuba diving is to learn to dive in a pool and, eventually, become certified divers. The Professional Association of Diving Instructors (PADI) offers more diver-certification courses than any other organization. PADI-certified instructors offer intro-to-scuba courses in most community swimming pools across the country.

The Basics

- The first step you and your kids must take to explore the sport of scuba diving is to learn to dive in a pool and, eventually, become certified divers.

- Introductory scuba diving courses are offered to kids beginning at age 8; children may become fully certified divers at age 10.

- The Florida Keys is the primary scuba diving destination in the continental US.

- Scuba equipment manufacturers are just introducing scuba gear sized specifically for children.

In recent years, PADI has made a concerted effort to introduce children to diving. The organization's Supplied-Air Snorkeling for Youth program is aimed at giving children younger than 8 a taste of scuba diving by using a floating air cylinder and breathing hose that enables young children to breathe "underwater" while swimming face down at the water's surface. Next, the association's Bubblemaker course gives 8- and 9-year-olds a true sense of underwater breathing.

PADI introduces scuba diving to children ages 8 and up through its Seal Team, an instruction program that teaches scuba through a series of "AquaMissions." Seal Team members learn to dive while playing with flashlights, taking pictures, and floating like astronauts underwater.

When they turn 10, kids may take PADI's Junior Scuba Diver and Junior Open Water courses, which lead to full diving certification. PADI also offers its Discover Scuba program to parents and children together at dive centers and destinations around the world.

For more information about certification or to find certification courses near you, go to www.padi.com. Also check with pools in your area to learn of other certified courses offered there.

Where to Scuba

If you think of scuba diving as primarily an international sport, you're right. But there are plenty of scuba diving destinations in the US for you and your kids to try out the sport affordably.

The Florida Keys comprise the primary scuba diving destination in the continental US. Hawaii is a top destination as well. In addition, clear lakes across the country offer decent diving possibilities. Be forewarned, however: If you and your kids really get hooked on diving, pricey trips to the coral reefs of the Caribbean, the South Pacific, and/or Australia may be in your future.

To find dive sites near your home, check out the map of US dive locations maintained by *Dive Training* magazine. Go to www.dtmag.com (keywords: Diving USA). In addition, the website www.shorediving.com lists hundreds of potential shore-access dive sites around the country, as recommended by divers and vetted by other divers.

The Florida Keys comprise the primary scuba diving destination in the continental US.

Scuba Gear for Kids

As with so many outdoor action sports, scuba equipment manufacturers are just introducing gear—in this case, underwater-breathing-apparatus rigs—sized specifically for children.

Scuba gear manufacturers Dive Rite (www.diverite.com) and Oceanic (www.oceanicworldwide.com) now offer **buoyancy compensators** and **regulators** for children. Dive Rite's kid-size buoyancy compensator comes with interchangeable straps so that one size fits children ages 10 to 16. The smallest Oceanic buoyancy compensator fits children who weigh as little as 55 pounds.

Small **cylinders**, or tanks, suitable for children are just reaching the market. Not all dive centers carry the small cylinders. If you find a dive center that has the cylinders in a location you'll be diving with your kids, be sure to reserve them in advance.

Because children long have been snorkeling, there are plenty of kid-size **masks**, **fins**, and **wetsuits** on the market. Many such kid-specific items are of low quality, however. If your children are big enough, you may want to outfit them with small women's gear instead.

Possibilities

JOHN PENNEKAMP CORAL REEF STATE PARK

Florida's John Pennekamp Coral Reef State Park encompasses 25 miles of coastline and almost 200 nautical square miles of ocean and coral reef at the eastern end of the Florida Keys near Key Largo. Pennekamp Park is the top diving destination in the contiguous US.

The park was established in 1963 as the country's first undersea preserve. Pennekamp protects the heart of the Florida Keys barrier reef, the only living coral reef in the continental US and the third longest in the world.

Located an hour's drive south of Miami, the park hosts more than a million visitors each year.

The John Pennekamp Institute of Scuba Diving (305-451-6322; www.pennekamppark.com) holds the concession for providing boat access, guided dives, and dive instruction in the park.

If you plan to camp at the park's campground, advance reservations are a must. For more information, visit www.floridastateparks.org/pennekamp.

FLORIDA KEYS NATIONAL MARINE SANCTUARY

In the decades after the creation of John Pennekamp Coral Reef State Park, ongoing degradation of the Florida Keys barrier reef convinced Congress to create the Florida Keys National Marine Sanctuary in 1990. The sanctuary's 2800 nautical square miles encompass the reef outside Pennekamp State Park's boundaries.

Visit www.fknms.nos.noaa.gov to learn more about the sanctuary, and then visit www.thefloridakeys.com/dive to

Shorediving.com

The website www.shorediving.com lists hundreds of potential shore-access dive sites around the country, as recommended by divers and vetted by other divers.

learn about the many diving opportunities the sanctuary presents and the dive centers that provide access to the reef's many dive locations.

HAWAII

Each of Hawaii's eight main islands is home to several diving hot spots. Diving in Hawaii features reefs of intense color and an incredible variety of sea life. Most diving is done off the islands' calmer leeward coasts, where visibility ranges to 100 feet.

Dive centers and charters are numerous and competitive on the islands. You'll need to troll information about the islands on the internet or check out Lonely Planet Publications' *Diving and Snorkeling Hawaii* by Casey and Astrid Mahaney to learn what Hawaiian dive locations most interest you. In addition, visit www.shorediving.com for descriptions of 80 possible Hawaiian shore dives.

Each of Hawaii's eight main islands is home to several diving hot spots.

LAKE OUACHITA

According to the Environmental Protection Agency, Lake Ouachita, located in west-central Arkansas, is the second clearest lake in the US. That fact—the result of the lake's undeveloped shoreline—makes Ouachita one of the better lake-diving locations in the country, with literally hundreds of potential dive sites.

Three area dive shops cater to Lake Ouachita divers. Visit www.shorediving.com for Ouachita diving details, and www.arkansasstateparks.com (Keywords: Lake Ouachita), for information about Lake Ouachita State Park.

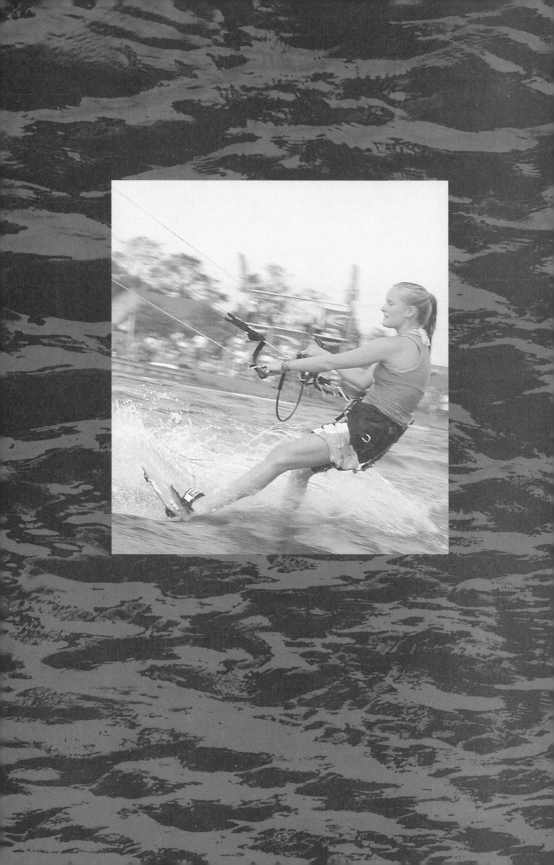

24 Kiteboarding

Kiteboarding, a sport that was invented in the 1980s and took off in the late 1990s, involves standing on a board and riding it across a body of water while being towed by a wind-borne, parachute-like kite. It may well be the hottest outdoor action sport among American youth today. (North Carolina-based Real Kiteboarding, the world's largest kiteboarding school, trained more than 6000 kiteboarders in 2005, double the number who took classes only two years earlier.)

Kids are flocking to kiteboarding because it offers everything they want in a sport: tremendous fun in the sun, a short (though steep) learning curve, affordability, and the opportunity to pull off high-adrenaline tricks like spins and backward rolls in a safe, flatwater environment.

Those same qualities make kiteboarding a great sport to try with your children, who are apt to take to the sport almost instantly. They may well become part of kiteboarding's youth vanguard taking the sport to new heights of athleticism. (As of this writing, the current Professional Kiteboard Riders Association Tour Champ is 16 years old, while the reigning men's Red Bull King of the Air—the sport's Super Bowl—is 17.)

Getting Started

Though competitive kiteboarding is ruled by youth these days, recreational kiteboarding is a great sport for parents and kids to take up together. Family classes are offered at most kiteboarding schools. Because kiteboarding demands more skill than many other outdoor action sports, most kiteboarding experts recommend that parents encourage their children to wait until they're 10 to take up the sport, and the minimum age for most kiteboarding school classes is 10 as well.

Kiteboarding schools offer introductory courses in kite flying through the use of practice kites that are simply small versions of the kites used for kiteboarding. These practice kites will enable you and your kids to get a jump on the sport before you take to the beach and water with full-size kites.

Practice kites also are available for purchase. Real Kiteboarding, for example, offers a package that includes a learning video and training kite for $100.

After you have your kite-flying skills down, you'll be ready for the half-day introductory courses as well as longer courses offered by kiteboarding schools that take students from beginner to self-sufficient intermediate kiteboarder in several intensive days.

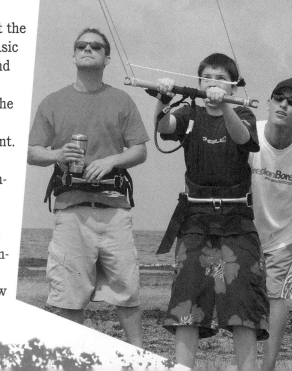

Once you've got the equipment and basic know-how, you and your kids will be ready to take to the water together whenever you want.

How much fun will you have coming into the sport as an adult? It's worth noting that famed world-champion windsurfer Robbie Naish, now in his mid-40s, has given up windsurfing for the outrageous fun of kiteboarding. And you can pretty much count on your kids liking the sport as well.

Trip Forman, who founded Real Kiteboarding with a partner in 1998, says many youngsters are taking up the sport today through their parents. "A lot of our former clients now have kids old enough to kiteboard," says Forman. "They come out and ride together every weekend—moms, dads, boys, girls, all sorts of family combinations."

Forman says virtually everyone who tries kiteboarding ends up loving the sport, especially kids. "The only thing they need to have is comfort in the water," he says. "I haven't seen one kid who hasn't liked it."

The Basics

- Kiteboarding may well be the hottest outdoor action sport among American youth today.

- Recreational kiteboarding is a great sport for parents and kids to take up together.

- The learning-to-kiteboard progression involves learning to fly a training kite, and then taking an introductory course at a beach.

- The entire country lends itself well to the sport of kiteboarding; all that's necessary is a small body of water and a bit of wind.

- Kid kiteboarders use the same gear small adults use in high winds.

As for where to ride, though many outdoor action sports are best practiced in the wide-open West, the East Coast—with its prevailing winds out of the west—makes for tremendous kiteboarding.

"I came to kiteboarding from other outdoor sports," says Forman. "This is the first outdoor sport I tried that didn't make me curse living on the East Coast. In fact, the East Coast is perfect for kiteboarding."

Indeed, says Forman, the entire country lends itself well to the sport.

"All you need is a little wind and any body of water," he says.

Michigan, Kansas, Georgia, Vermont, Texas, Indiana, and any other state not normally associated with outdoor action sports, all are loaded with potential kiteboarding sites.

Possibilities

REAL KITEBOARDING

Like kayaking, rock climbing, and other gear- and skill-intensive outdoor action sports, kiteboarding is best tackled with the help of instructors.

"In the spring of 1998, I learned to kiteboard on my own because there wasn't anybody teaching," says Real Kiteboarding owner Trip Forman. "I wouldn't wish that experience on my worst enemy. Without instruction, kiteboarding gear is useless. It's like owning a plane and not knowing how to fly."

Cape Hatteras, North Carolina-based Real Kiteboarding, named by *Outside* magazine as one of the top 10 adventure camps in the world, is the clear leader in kiteboarding instruction today.

Forman attributes his young staff's skill and enthusiasm for the sport as one reason for the center's top-dog status. Another reason, says Forman, is Real Kiteboarding's location on North Carolina's Outer Banks. Pamlico Sound, the stretch of water between the state's coast and its outer-rim islands, is a great spot to learn to kiteboard.

"The sound is like a huge practice pool," says Forman. "Thirty-five miles in every direction of waist-deep, flat water. Plus, the waves are terrific on the ocean side of the Banks."

Real Kiteboarding's three-day Zero to Hero beginner camp runs $900. The school will arrange a three-day family camp for $1000 per family member.

North Carolina's Outer Banks offer a great opportunity to combine a family getaway with a chance to learn to kiteboard. Camping is available, or vacation homes can be rented by the week.

"You can go to the beach, learn to kiteboard, have bonfires on the shore at night," says Forman. "It's really the perfect family vacation."

For more information about Real Kiteboarding, call 866-732-5548 or go to www.realkiteboarding.com.

> "Without instruction, kiteboarding gear is useless," says Trip Forman. "It's like owning a plane and not knowing how to fly."

SOUTH PADRE ISLAND KITEBOARDING

Like North Carolina's Outer Banks, the calm water between the coast and long, sandy South Padre Island at the south tip of Texas provides great conditions for kiteboarding.

South Padre Island Kiteboarding is the only dedicated kiteboarding school on the island. As with Real Kiteboarding, South Padre Island Kiteboarding offers a variety of classes and camps aimed at budding boarders of all ages, including families. Costs range from $75 for an introductory class in kite flying to $1200 for a four-day, one-on-one immersion course.

For more information, call 956-245-8343 or visit www.southpadreislandkiteboarding.com.

HOOD RIVER WATERPLAY

Hood River WaterPlay offers a Kids Kite Kamp on the same stretch of the Columbia River famous for windsurfing. The same upstream winds that make the Columbia River Gorge terrific for windsurfing make the spot great for learning to kiteboard as well.

The Oregon school's Kids Kite Kamp is open to children weighing a minimum of 85 pounds. Alternatively, you and your children can take a course together. Hood River's 90-minute introductory course costs $85 per person, while combined morning and afternoon courses range from $250 to $400.

For more information, call 541-386-9463 or visit www.hoodriverwaterplay.com.

WEST COAST KITEBOARDING

West Coast Kiteboarding is based in San Diego, where conditions are not as optimal for kiteboarding as on the East Coast because the open Pacific waters are rough, and winds usually blow directly out of the west onto the north-south San Diego beach. Still, West Coast Kiteboarding offers on-beach kite instruction at its San Diego site, along with on-water instruction when conditions permit. The company also offers land and water instruction at its protected-water, side-wind beach site 200 miles south of San Diego in San Quintin, Baja California, Mexico.

Half- and full-day lessons cost from $170 to $300. For more information, call 619-813-2230 or visit www.westcoastkiteboarding.com.

SNOW KITEBOARDING

If your kids are into snowboarding but you're not into the whole resort-based snowboarding scene, snow kiteboarding may be the answer for you.

Snow kiteboarding enables snowboarders to ride by harnessing wind energy.

Rather than using lifts and gravity to ride, snow kiteboarding enables snowboarders to ride by harnessing wind energy. The idea of strapping on a snowboard, latching onto a kite, and taking off across a snow-covered field or frozen, snow-covered lake is new, but Real Kiteboarding's Trip Forman says he believes the sport may eventually grow bigger than water kiteboarding.

Forman says the fun he had the first winter he tried snow kiteboarding told him all he needed to know about the sport's potential. "I got fully hooked," he says. "I rode more than 40 days in Vermont, New Hampshire, New York, Ohio, Indiana, and Michigan. I didn't buy one lift ticket—and I canceled my planned heli-ski trip. I got so much powder I didn't need it."

Real Kiteboarding now offers snow kiteboarding instruction during the winter months in Madison, Wisconsin; Lake Winnipesaukee, New Hampshire; Burlington, Vermont; and Summit County, Colorado.

Kiteboarding Gear for Kids

Unlike other outdoor action sports, kiteboarding gear suitable for kids has been available since the sport's inception. And, says Real Kiteboarding owner Trip Forman: "It's not just Mickey Mouse stuff either. It's all the same gear. Kids just use smaller kites than adults, that's all."

In addition to kites, lines, **harnesses**, and boards, to go kiteboarding you and your kids will need **PFDs**, **helmets** (hockey helmets are most common), and, depending on weather and water conditions, **wetsuits** and **booties**.

These days, most **kiteboarding kites** are inflatable. That means they have a leading edge that holds air and keeps them "powered up" and ready for relaunch after falls.

Most **kiteboarding boards** are bidirectional, or twin-tip. The boarder's feet remain in the board's two straps, and the boarder simply switches from riding toe down to riding heel down when jibing, or changing directions.

New, a full kiteboard setup costs between $1500 and $3000. But kiteboarding has been around long enough now that you'll be able to find used and closeout gear on the market for yourself and your kids. Even so, you'll still be looking at several hundred dollars for each full kiteboard setup you purchase.

Shopping for kid kiteboarding gear is easier than for other outdoor sport kid gear because kids simply use small adult gear. Big-name kiteboarding gear manufacturers worth checking out include Wipika (www.wipikakiteboarding.com), Liquid Force (www.liquidforcekites.com), and Naish (www.naishkites.com).

Kiteboards and kites are designed to be transported in carriers roughly the size of golf-club bags, making them easy and free to check on commercial flights.

Check *Kiteboarding* magazine's website, www.kiteboardingmag.com, for more information on kiteboarding and kiteboarding gear. In addition, go to www.kitesurfingschool.org for a good kiteboarding overview and an online used-gear marketplace.

Resources

Extreme and Not-so-Extreme Dayhiking

ORGANIZATIONS AND OUTFITTERS

Sharing Nature Foundation: www.sharingnature.com

Geocaching—The Official GPS Global Cache Hunt Site:
www.geocaching.com

US Orienteering Federation: www.us.orienteering.org

Learn Orienteering: www.learn-orienteering.org

Trail Runner magazine: www.trailrunnermag.com

GEAR

GPS rental units from Lower Gear: 480-767-1874;
www.lowergear.com

Kid running shoes from New Balance: 800-253-7463;
www.newbalance.com

BOOKS

Sharing Nature with Children: By Joseph Cornell, Dawn
Publications 1998

Sharing Nature with Children II: By Joseph Cornell, Dawn
Publications 1989

Trail Runner's Guide: San Diego: By Jerry Schad,
Wilderness Press 2004

Trail Runner's Guide: San Francisco Bay Area: By Jessica Lage,
Wilderness Press 2003

Peak Bagging

ORGANIZATIONS AND OUTFITTERS

Highpointers Club: www.highpointers.org

LOCALES

Mt. Tamalpais, California: www.mttam.net

Gettysburg National Military Park, Pennsylvania:
www.nps.gov/gett

Piestewa Peak, Arizona: www.phoenix.gov/parks
(keyword: Piestewa)

Grays and Torreys peaks, Colorado: www.14ers.com

Mt. Sneffels, Colorado: www.14ers.com

Mt. Jefferson, New Hampshire: www.fs.fed.us
(keywords: White Mountain)

Springer Mountain, Georgia: www.georgiatrails.com

Mt. St. Helens, Washington: www.fs.fed.us/gpnf

GEAR

Colorado Fourteener pins from Top Peak: 888-297-4474;
www.toppeak.com

BOOKS

Colorado's Fourteeners: By Gerry Roach,
Fulcrum Publishing 1999

Canyoneering

ORGANIZATIONS AND OUTFITTERS

Zion Adventure Company: 435-772-0990; www.zionadventures.com

LOCALES

Zion Canyon Narrows, Utah: www.nps.gov/zion

Peek-a-Boo, Spooky, and Brimstone canyons, Utah:
www.canyoneeringusa.com/utah/esca/drycoy.htm

Water Holes Canyon, Arizona:
www.americansouthwest.net/slot_canyons

Buckskin Gulch, Utah: www.americansouthwest.net/slot_canyons

Fern Canyon, California: www.redwoodvisitor.org (keywords: Fern
Canyon); or Prairie Redwoods State Park, 707-464-6101

Aravaipa Canyon, Arizona: www.recreation.gov (keyword:
Aravaipa); Bureau of Land Management, 928-348-4400

Panthertown Valley, North Carolina: www.hikinginthesmokies.com

King's Canyon and Yosemite Valley, California: www.nps.gov/seki
and www.nps.gov/yose

Havasu Canyon, Arizona: www.havasupaitribe.com

GEAR

Canyoneering shoes from Five.Ten: 909-798-4222;
www.fiveten.com

Backpacking

LOCALES

Isle au Haut, Acadia National Park, Maine: www.nps.gov/acad

Angel Island, San Francisco Bay, California: www.angelisland.org

Orcas Island, San Juan Islands, Washington:
www.orcasisland.org

Little River Valley, Van Damme State Park, California:
www.parks.ca.gov (keywords: Van Damme)

Johnson Creek Recreation Area, Shawnee National Forest,
Illinois: www.fs.fed.us (keyword: Shawnee)

Grand Canyon National Park, Arizona: www.nps.gov/grca

Canyonlands National Park, Utah: www.nps.gov/cany

Pinkham Notch to Tuckerman Ravine, Mt. Washington, New
Hampshire: www.tuckerman.org

Appalachian Trail, Georgia to Maine: www.appalachiantrail.org

Yosemite National Park, California: www.nps.gov/yose

Glacier National Park, Montana: www.nps.gov/glac

Yellowstone National Park, Wyoming: www.nps.gov/yell

Shenandoah National Park, Virginia: www.nps.gov/shen

Pacific Crest Trail, southern Sierra portion, California:
www.pcta.org

Long Trail, Vermont: www.greenmountainclub.org

John Muir Trail, California: www.pcta.org

Cirque of the Towers, Wind River Mountains, Wyoming:
www.visitsublettecounty.com

Colorado Trail, Colorado: www.coloradotrail.org

Continental Divide Trail, Colorado: www.cdtrail.org

Grand Gulch Primitive Area, Utah: www.ut.blm.gov/monticello

Wonderland Trail, Mt. Ranier National Park, Washington:
www.nps.gov/mora

Denali National Park, Alaska: www.nps.gov/dena

Backpacking Made Easier:
Llama Trekking and Hut Trips

ORGANIZATIONS AND OUTFITTERS

Llama information: www.llama.org

English Mountain Llama Treks, North Carolina: 828-622-9686;
www.hikinginthesmokies.com

Wild Earth Llama Adventures, New Mexico: 800-758-5262;
   www.llamaadventures.com
Appalachian Mountain Club huts, New Hampshire:
   603-466-2727; www.outdoors.org/lodging/huts
10th Mountain Division Hut Association, Colorado:
   970-925-5775; www.huts.org

Mountain Biking

ORGANIZATIONS AND OUTFITTERS
New England Mountain Bike Association: www.nemba.org
International Mountain Bicycling Association: www.imba.com
Freeriding information: www.mtb-freeride.com
Mountain Bike Hall of Fame: www.mtnbikehalloffame.com
Western Spirit Cycling Adventures: 800-845-2453;
   www.westernspirit.com

LOCALES
Moab, Utah: www.discovermoab.com
White Rim Trail, Canyonlands National Park, Utah:
   www.nps.gov/cany
Crested Butte, Colorado: www.visitcrestedbutte.com
Mountain biking meccas-on-the-make: www.mbronline.com
   (keyword: Destinations); www.gorp.away.com
   (keywords: Beyond Moab)
West Virginia: www.bicyclewv.com
New River Gorge, West Virginia: www.nps.gov/neri
Monongahela National Forest, West Virginia: www.fs.fed.us
   (keyword: Monongahela)
Bend, Oregon: www.visitbend.com
Sun Valley, Idaho: www.visitsunvalley.com
Custer, South Dakota: www.custersd.com
Park City, Utah: www.parkcityinfo.com
Durango, Colorado: www.durango.org

Bouldering and Roped Rock Climbing

ORGANIZATIONS AND OUTFITTERS
Rock climbing information: www.rockclimbing.com;
   www.climbing.com
Bouldering information: www.bouldering.com;
   www.newenglandbouldering.com

273

High Angle Adventures: 800-777-2546, www.highangle.com

Eastern Mountain Sports Climbing School: 800-310-4504;
www.emsclimb.com

Mountain Adventure Seminars: 209-753-6556;
www.mtadventure.com

LOCALES

Joshua Tree National Park, California: www.nps.gov/jotr

Muir Valley, Kentucky: www.muirvalley.com

GEAR

Kid climbing shoes by EB: www.eb-france.com

Kid climbing shoes by Montrail: www.montrail.com

Kid climbing shoes by Five.Ten: www.fiveten.com

Kid climbing helmet by Edelrid: www.edelrid.de

Kid climbing harness by Trango: www.trango.com

Kid climbing harness by Black Diamond: www.bdel.com

BOOKS

New England Bouldering: By Tim Kemple,
Wolverine Publishing 2004

Backcountry Skiing

ORGANIZATIONS AND OUTFITTERS

Telemark skiing information: www.telemarkski.com

LOCALES

Portneuf Range Yurt System, Idaho: 208-282-2945;
www.isu.edu/outdoor (keyword: yurts)

Sierra Club huts, California: 800-679-6775; www.sierraclub.org
(keyword: huts)

10th Mountain Division Hut Association, Colorado:
970-925-5775; www.huts.org

GEAR

Kid telemark skis by Karhu: www.karhu.com

Kid telemark skis by K2: www.k2skis.com

Kid telemark boots by Garmont: www.garmont.com

Climbing skins by Black Diamond: www.bdel.com

Climbing skins by Backcountry Access: www.bcaccess.com

Climbing skins by G3: www.genuineguidegear.com

River Running

ORGANIZATIONS AND OUTFITTERS
Nantahala Outdoor Center: 888-905-7238; www.noc.com
Zoar Outdoor: 800-532-7483; www.zoaroutdoor.com
Canyon REO: 800-272-3353; www.canyonreo.com
OARS: 800-346-6277; www.oars.com

GEAR
River gear online retailer NRS: www.nrsweb.com
River gear online retailer Riversports: www.riversports.com
Boat manufacturer Aire: www.aire.com
Boat manufacturer Jack's Plastic Welding: www.jpwinc.com
Boat manufacturer Hyside: www.hyside.com
Boat manufacturer Star: www.starinflatables.com

Whitewater Kayaking

ORGANIZATIONS AND OUTFITTERS
Whitewater kayak schools: www.wavelengthmagazine.com;
   www.paddlermagazine.com (keyword: Tripfinder)
Zoar Outdoor: 800-532-7483; www.zoaroutdoor.com
Nantahala Outdoor Center: 888-905-7238; www.noc.com
Sundance River Center: 888-777-7557; www.sundanceriver.com
Canyon Rio: 800-272-3353; www.canyonrio.com
List of whitewater parks: www.swwparkalliance.com
   (keywords: Whitewater Parks Around the Globe)
List of Wild and Scenic Rivers: www.nps.gov/rivers
   (keywords: Designated WSRs)

GEAR
Kid kayaks and paddles by Jackson Kayak:
   www.jacksonkayak.com
Kid drytops and personal flotation devices by Lotus Designs:
   www.lotusdesigns.com
Kid kayak helmets by Grateful Heads: www.gratefulheads.com
Kid kayak helmets by Shred Ready: www.shredready.com

Flatwater Canoeing and Sea Kayaking

ORGANIZATIONS AND OUTFITTERS
Williams and Hall Wilderness Guides and Outfitters:
   800-322-5837; www.williamsandhall.com

Boundary Waters Canoe Area Wilderness permit and quota
information: www.bwcaw.org
Tex's Riverway Adventures: 435-259-5101; www.texsriverways.com
Discovery Sea Kayaks: 360-378-2559; www.discoveryseakayaks.com
Maine Island Kayak Company: 800-796-2373;
www.maineislandkayak.com

LOCALES
Apostle Islands National Lakeshore, Wisconsin:
www.nps.gov/apis

GEAR
Boundary Waters maps by Fisher Maps: www.fishermaps.com

BOOKS
Boundary Waters Canoe Area, Volumes 1 and 2:
By Robert Beymer, Wilderness Press 2000
Kayaking Puget Sound, the San Juans, and Gulf Islands:
By Randel Washburne and R. Carey Gersten,
Mountaineers Books 1999

Bodyboarding and Surfing

ORGANIZATIONS AND OUTFITTERS
International Bodyboarding Association pro tour:
www.ibatour.com
Surf tracking: www.surfline.com; www.surfinfo.com;
www.wannasurf.com; www.globalsurfers.com
Corolla Surf School: 252-453-9283; www.corollasurfshop.com
Wrightsville Beach Surf Camp: 866-844-7873; www.wbsurfcamp.com

LOCALES
Corolla, North Carolina: www.outerbanks.com/corolla

BOOKS
The Stormrider Guide: North America: By Drew Kampion,
Low Pressure Publications 2002

Scuba Diving

ORGANIZATIONS AND OUTFITTERS
Map of US dive locations: www.dtmag.com
(keywords: Diving USA)

Professional Association of Diving Instructors: 800-729-7234;
www.padi.com

List of US shore-access dive locations: www.shorediving.com

John Pennekamp Institute of Scuba Diving: 305-451-6322;
www.pennekamppark.com

Florida Keys dive locations: www.thefloridakeys.com/dive

LOCALES

John Pennekamp Coral Reef State Park, Florida:
www.floridastateparks.org/pennekamp

Florida Keys National Marine Sanctuary, Florida:
www.fknms.nos.noaa.gov

Lake Ouachita State Park, Arkansas:
www.arkansasstateparks.com (keywords: Lake Ouachita)

GEAR

Kid buoyancy compensators and regulators by Dive Rite:
www.diverite.com

Kid buoyancy compensators and regulators by Oceanic:
www.oceanicworldwide.com

BOOKS

Diving and Snorkeling Hawaii: By Casey Mahaney,
Lonely Planet Publications 2000

Kiteboarding

ORGANIZATIONS AND OUTFITTERS

Kiteboarding information: www.kiteboardingmag.com;
www.kitesurfingschool.org

Real Kiteboarding: 866-732-5548; www.realkiteboarding.com

South Padre Island Kiteboarding: 956-245-8343;
www.southpadreislandkiteboarding.com

Hood River Waterplay: 541-386-9463; www.hoodriverwaterplay.com

West Coast Kiteboarding: 619-813-2230;
www.westcoastkiteboarding.com

GEAR

Kiteboarding gear by Wipika:
www.wipikakiteboarding.com

Kiteboarding gear by Liquid Force:
www.liquidforcekites.com

Kiteboarding gear by Naish: www.naishkites.com

Index

About the Author

Scott Graham is the author of three previous outdoor/travel books, *Backpacking and Camping in the Developing World* (Wilderness Press), *Adventure Travel in Latin America* (Wilderness Press), and *Handle With Care: A Guide to Responsible Travel in Developing Countries* (Noble Press). He also wrote, with a co-author, *Coaching Six-and-Under Soccer: A Baffled Parent's Guide* (McGraw-Hill).

Graham lives with his wife, an emergency physician, and two sons in Durango, Colorado, where he and his family pursue outdoor action sports that include dayhiking, backpacking, rock climbing, mountain biking, kayaking, rafting, and skiing.

Photo Credits

All photos are by **Scott Graham**, except for the following:

GirlVentures (www.girlventures.org): ii (bottom left), 2, 33, 48, 60, 130, 146, 164, 190, 193, 194, 234, 244

Jackson Kayak (www.jacksonkayak.com): vi (Dane and Emily) 63, 208 (bottom middle and top), 222, 256

Professional Association of Diving Instructors (www.padi.com): 51, 90, 94, 260

REAL Kiteboarding (www.realkiteboarding.com): 208 (bottom right), 262, 264, 267, 269

Eric Pierson: vi (Carly), 160

Stuart Saslow: 196, 203, 207

Dana Siekman: xiv, 36, 58, 208 (bottom left), 246, 248, 251, 252, 254, 255

Mike White: 167

Caroline Winnett: 187 (top), 200

Nick Wilkes, Zion Adventure Company (www.zionadventures.com): 104 (bottom left), 137, 141